To Tom

my Life long Friend

May good HEALTH +
prosperity follow you
Always!

Stephen F Fugg

DON'T ASK ME HOW I FEEL

HOW I FEEL

I Have MS

BY

STEPHEN KNAPP

authorHOUSE®

AuthorHouse™
1663 Liberty Drive, Suite 200
Bloomington, IN 47403
www.authorhouse.com
Phone: 1-800-839-8640

This book is a work of non-fiction. Unless otherwise noted, the author and the publisher make no explicit guarantees as to the accuracy of the information contained in this book and in some cases, names of people and places have been altered to protect their privacy.

First published by AuthorHouse   10/21/2008

ISBN: 978-1-4389-0055-1 (e)
ISBN: 978-1-4389-0054-4 (sc)

Printed in the United States of America
Bloomington, Indiana

This book is printed on acid-free paper.

To my family

"YOU HAVE MULTIPLE Sclerosis and looking at your MRI, you are a walking time bomb. You may not have symptoms today, but it's just a matter of time." – Dr. Sonia Nunez, Neurologist, 10/22/2002.

Prior to my diagnosis I had no idea what Multiple Sclerosis was. No one in my family has ever had it. Much like so many other illnesses with long names, if I did not know someone who had it, I probably did not know anything about it. But, when something catches my attention, I delve into it full steam ahead. I will never consider myself an expert on MS. I am not a doctor. However, I have read a number of books about MS, I have attended many MS seminars, I have read extensively about it from ubiquitous internet sources, devoured all the pamphlets put out by the National Multiple Sclerosis Society, and other national organizations, and I have viewed videos on various subjects related to MS. I have also joined several local support groups who meet on a monthly basis. I now feel I have at least a fair degree of formal understanding about MS.

Moreover, I have a very personal and experiential understanding of the disease that one can only acquire by actually having MS.

The cause of MS is unknown. Some have suggested it is precipitated by environmental factors. Some say it may be caused by exposure to a virus. Others point to head trauma as a possible source. There is evidence to show it may have several causes, or come from several different predispositions. With the body research collected thus far on this topic, none of the above could be ruled out for me.

Multiple Sclerosis typically shows up in people between ages 20 to 40. To a lesser extent it can be found in children and people in their 50's or older. Recent research has been found which suggests that the cognitive effects of MS may begin at a very young age and only much later on develop into a more full range of physical and cognitive symptoms. This is the foundation for the major premise of this book.

MS affects each person differently and yet there are often clusters of characteristics that many of us with the disease all have at one time or another. It is impossible for you to feel what I feel. It is difficult for me to explain to you how I feel, especially if you have never felt the same things. The matter is further complicated by the fact proper vocabulary does not exist for many of the sensations that MS produces. Accurate and generally understandable and agreed upon names for them may not exist.

I am sure that no one who has MS will feel exactly all the things I feel in the same way I feel them. MS is like snowflakes, no two are exactly like. I have read enough to know there are similarities which many MS folks share. However, suffice it to say that everyone is unique and the full gamut of MS symptoms for any two people is likely to have some which are common to both, and some which may be completely different.

Imagine you have traveled alone to a foreign country. You eat something that makes you horribly sick. You try to get everyone's and anyone's attention but no one listens. You try to talk to them to say how you feel, but since you don't speak a language that they understand, they just look at you funny, like you are making it up or they think it's just in your head. You get frustrated that no one understands you, or believes you. Finally, you do find someone who thinks they get the message, or you find a doctor that seems to believe you, but what he diagnoses and prescribes for you is the wrong thing and it doesn't help. You feel awful, exasperated, and hopeless. You don't know which way to turn. You can't find anyone who can provide a solution or offer an explanation as to why you feel so badly. You've never had this before. No one you know has it. You get the feeling you are all alone with an unsolvable problem, and there is no one to turn to for help.

Now I've just described what it's like to have MS, except food poisoning doesn't usually last a lifetime. MS does.

Here's another way of looking at it. Imagine a large fleet of cars, hundreds of them, some are ten years old, some are twenty or thirty years old, or older. Let's say they all have MS (mechanical stress). They run sluggish. Some parts don't work right. Some parts make terrible noises or they smell bad.

The first technician looks at it and says "needs new spark plugs and points." The next one says, "Just needs more air pressure in the tires. The next one says its "faulty gas." The next one says, "Trust me. It needs a complete diagnostic check and a full tune-up."

Ka-ching. Ka-ching.

You are now confused, you've paid lots of money, and the car still runs with no zip. And no one has the answer.

This is somewhat like person with MS who desperately needs someone to tell them what's going on. But, to no avail, this only contributes to more confusion and frustration.

Characteristically, MS produces feelings that we call "tingly" or "numbness" or "burning sensation." Some MS symptoms may involve paralysis, or restricted movement, or pain, or fatigue, or spasms, or tremors, or visual problems and a host of others. Prior to my diagnosis these words did not carry the same definitions that they now do for me. This is because they all represent physical sensations that I have felt, and having felt them as associated with MS, they are now quite different. For example, MS pain is different than other kinds of pain. MS fatigue is different than other kinds of fatigue, and so on down the list.

This is because they all represent physical sensations that I have felt, and having personally felt them as associated with MS, they are emphatically different. The word "freezing" has a certain dictionary founded definition, but being in ten below zero temperatures, standing on snowy ground, feeling the wind bite your skin and nip your ears with excruciatingly pain and your toes becoming so numb you can't feel them. This kind of freezing is much different than the word on the page may imply.

In the same way, all the MS symptoms I just mentioned are different because I have been there, done that, had them over and over again. You don't know freezing until you've really been out there in freezing temperatures, aching, shivering, or weakening. I didn't know MS until long after I had it, and knew what kinds of things it does to a body. The MS words take on a whole new meaning when you've been there.

For example, MS pain is different than other kinds of pain. MS fatigue is different than other kinds of fatigue, and so on down the list. When I speak from a position of having MS I can contrast the feelings I have now with those feelings I had earlier in my life. I was accustomed to having a range of "normal" feelings that probably all other normal people will agree on when applying the same terms because they are quite familiar. The feelings I have now are a new set which are felt by only a relatively small number of people, men and women, young and old alike, who have MS. The terms we use for these feelings may sound familiar to others without the disease, but they have no idea what we are feeling when we express ourselves in these terms. And, to be sure, the terms not only have a physical element to each of them, but they also are charged with psychological and cognitive issues as well. Furthermore, to make things even more complicated, most MS feelings occur on the inside of our bodies, invisible to us and to all others.

Having said all of that, I have attempted to describe many of the MS-related feelings, thoughts, and reactions that I have experienced. I have shared some of these with others who have MS and the comments they have replied back to me in return were very positive. I have hit a lot of things right on the head in my descriptions. Those out there who have some form of MS responded by saying I have succinctly captured what they felt but were not able to put these feelings into words.

Being reinforced by their comments I have been compelled to take them further. These have now become my goals. I first want to tell those who are unfamiliar with MS what it is like. What it feels like to have MS, and how it affects our lives. Secondly, for those who do have it, or think they may have it, I want them to know what I know. I want to explain in vivid detail what I have felt, so that they may be more enlightened and less frightened. It is unbelievably scary to think you are the only one who feels this way. It is of great comfort to realize there are many who share similar kinds of strange feelings. Finally, I want to share some of the problems I have had to face and elaborate on how I approached solving them. I feel far better today than I did two years ago, and it is not an accident.

There is an old saying that there are only three kinds of people – the ones who make things happen, the ones who let things happen, and the ones who don't realize that anything is happening. In the last year and a half I have journeyed through all three stages. I am still traveling in time towards new experiences, new information, new research findings and new treatments. I am attuned to my body now, and I "listen" to it speak to me through its physical responses. I am far from understanding the dynamics, and the cause – and - effect relationships, pertaining to each physical sensation, but I am much further down the path of knowledge about MS than where I began years ago.

This book has developed from periodic changes in my condition which has given me many physical and cognitive experiences to write about. As you will read later, I have had MS since early childhood. The symptoms that I had during the majority of my life were annoying and bothersome at times, more damaging than I could have ever known and often invisible. They were disguised in their cognitive characteristics, to the extent, or severity, that I never even knew I had anything. I thought I was mostly quite normal.

The things that made me different I discounted as inconsequential. I did get strange looks from others occasionally, which made me wonder, but I discounted them completely.

Actually, I considered myself superior physically and mentally in a number of ways. I was an outstanding junior golfer who tied a course record at age 14. I played basketball, football, and golf on school teams in starting positions in junior and senior high school. I was a good swimmer and diver. I was even city champion of a marble tournament in grade school. I was decent at tennis, ping pong, and badminton. I was a fast runner, too.

I was endowed with great physical stamina and required little sleep. As I was completing my final year of high school I passed all the physical requirements to be admitted to the United States Air Force Academy. And I made good grades.

When the USAF dream became short-lived I played golf on a scholarship at Utah State University, in Logan, Utah. After graduating from college with a double major BS in Psychology and Sociology, I became a member of the PGA. Nine years later I changed careers and for nearly three years I attended college, at the University of Houston at Clear Lake City, TX. I received an MBA, Masters Degree in Business Administration and Marketing took 30 hours of accounting and 9 hours of Labor Relations; worked 48 hours per week on a rotating shift at a chemical plant, and flew home and back every month for four days to see my family in Kansas. I averaged approximately 4 hours of sleep per night, or day, for all of that time. I made excellent grades. I never got sick or had to see a doctor. Nine years later while working full time, but then living with my family, I earned a second masters degree (MPA, Masters in Public Administration) taking night classes at Florida Atlantic University, in Boca Raton, Florida, earning a 3.7 GPA. Even though I didn't play nearly as often, I could still hit the golf ball well, with drives sometimes over 300 yards, and scored close to par when I had the chance to play.

I ask - Does that sound like someone who has a disease? How could I have a neurological disease? Could I have suspected I had a disabling disease that affects both the body and the mind in many different ways? Could anyone have known I was housing a disease in my body? I was active, happy, enjoying my family, making a living working hard toward retirement and was ostensibly healthy. Having an incurable disease inside of me was beyond my comprehension. Not me. Impossible, so I thought.

At this point I will pass on a thought that I have mentioned to others. Having MS, and no doubt many other diseases are equally applicable, is like being a member of a very exclusive club. You have to have it to be a member because members speak a language not understood by non-members. MS club members have a unique perspective based on personal experience which cannot possibly be fully understood or empathized by those who are on the outside.

All members share a common bond which ties them forever to each other. It is a bond of understanding. It's an esoteric connection that keeps us from feeling alone. It's a belonging and familiarity that places us all on the same side of the fence. I have been a member of this club for a very long time. I just didn't know it.

THE EARLY YEARS

1

MY NAME IS Stephen Foxall Knapp. I was destined to be the proverbial All American Boy. I had everything going for me. I had every possible reason to succeed with every impediment meticulously removed to insure a wonderfully fantastic life. Strangely, things did not go nearly as well as they should have. No one had any idea what or who was responsible for the horrendous barrage of unpredictable mis-steps, egregiously poor decisions, inexplicable periods of low achievement, and manifest behaviors shockingly embarrassing to family and friends.

Folks in Coffeyville, Kansas, just shrugged their shoulders and woefully wagged their heads in disbelief. Nothing made sense, but there it was, plain as day. There was talent and intelligence, to be sure, but gone awry for no apparent reason. There were signs of potential stemming from solid roots and a long heritage of honor and pride and success in the family linage. Something made no sense. But, what?

"That Stevie Knapp, he's a one of a kind, all right. He's a good boy, smart as a whip. Just can't quite put my finger on it, but there's something there that isn't quite right." – Mrs. Harris, his First Grade teacher, Edgewood Elementary School, Coffeyville, Kansas.

I was a walking enigma, and clueless as to why. I've had MS all my life and just didn't know how to read the signs. But, then, no one else did either.

My grandmother Knapp once told me a story about my father when he was about 10. He was playing hide and seek with the neighborhood kids running all around everywhere, getting dirty, hot and sweaty. The year was 1929, and they were living in a small Kansas community.

Mrs. Johnston hollered "Get out of them there bushes!" Mrs. Johnston, an elderly, gray-haired woman with a voice that sounded like fingernails scratching a black board, lived next door but was never a friendly sort." Get out of them there bushes or I'll take a switch to you, Charles. You hear me?" She spent most of her life hiding behind the dark green shades of her living room window, or peeking out the back screened-in door and rarely came outside.

My Dad said, "Is that, uh, proper, Mother, quoting her - them, there bushes?"

"No, son, it's not. But, heh, heh, that's all right. Don't worry your head off about it. She don't know no better."

In one way of thinking that just about sums up my whole life. I have been plodding along for well over 50 years and I just don't know no better. Still.

My story begins before I was born. My parents, Charles and Elizabeth Knapp married in 1945, in Indianapolis, Indiana. Mom was helping with the Red Cross war efforts and happened to get a blind date with a nice looking young Naval officer. She was a soft spoken, sophisticated, pretty blue-eyed blonde. The attraction was instantaneous.

WWII pulled Dad out into the South Pacific, but they kept in close contact. During the war Dad put his time in on ships and submarines, and then went back for the Korean War. It wasn't until four years after they tied the knot that they had their first Baby Boomer – a boy they named Stephen Foxall Knapp.

Charles and Betty had every reason to expect their son was going to be a huge success at something someday. My Dad was a brilliant young man with a high IQ who was making a name for himself as an officer, and had his own bright future in front of him.

My mother was well bred, coming from a fine lineage, educated, groomed, well-connected socially, a daughter of the American Revolution, a member of the Colonial Dames. She was very beautiful with a petite trim figure. Her father was an engineer with Link Belt, and her mother was a member of many social clubs, and a generous benefactor to many local Indianapolis and national organizations.

Charles had been very successful in his high school years. He was a drum major, valedictorian of his class and played Starting Guard on his high school basketball team. He earned a degree in journalism from the University of Michigan. He enlisted and eventually became a Rear Admiral in the US Navy. His specialty was submarines. He must have liked them because we have a slew of submarine pictures, more than you could shake a stick at, framed and hanging on the walls of many of the rooms in our house including my bedroom.

We also have an amazing board with about a hundred different hand-tied knots displayed on it and a picture of six submarines floating beside a big naval ship. Dad told me it was a present from his crew, a token of appreciation, when he left. They must have liked him a lot to spend that much time making it.

Mom said he really liked the discipline in the Navy. I later thought this was odd as he wasn't particularly disciplined in his family growing up. Clearly, he was not very strict with me.

He returned from WWII and attended the University of Kansas. He was cum laud in his law class and completed his JD degree in a year and a half. He was recalled back to the Navy for the Korean War, and his desire was to be a naval attorney remaining in the service as a legal officer for his career. His father, my grandfather, Dallas Knapp, secretly withheld his re-enlistment application until after the deadline.

My father's idea of his career path, remain in the Navy, was abruptly changed to join his Dad and formed the partnership Knapp and Knapp Attorneys, Coffeyville, Kansas. "Sonny," that's what he called Dad. "You are going to go to work for me. I need you here while I go back and forth to Topeka. You look after things here." He smiled and nodded his head persuasively up and down as he spoke.

Grandfather Knapp, though very well thought of and highly respected locally and as a state senator for 16 years, treated my Dad with very little respect and the partnership never really prospered. One year my grandfather even ran for the US Senate, but he didn't win.

He worked closely with Alf Lamdon, governor of Kansas, and presidential candidate who ran against FDR. Our lives would be much different if he'd won. But that's just the way the cookie crumbles.

I never felt like I knew Grandfather Knapp very well. He was a large man and all my remembrances of him were when he was sitting down in a comfortable chair or eating a meal.

Dad had one sister, Mary, who married Frank Liebert, who also was an attorney in Coffeyville, with his brother, Richard. Uncle Frank told me a story about my grandfather, years after Dallas had passed away......

"Hello, Dallas. How's every thing these days in your neck of the woods?" Will Rogers, renowned cowboy, businessman, broadcaster, and writer, dressed in jeans and a blue cattle bridge shirt with a red bandana tied around his neck had entered the law office on the second floor of the Terminal Building in downtown Coffeyville, Kansas.

There was nothing fancy or high flying about his law office. It was on the second story and was built entirely with wooden flooring. There were many wooden steps to climb, aided by a wooden rail to hang on to, and past the top of the stairs was a wooden door. Inside the door were lengths of wooden bookcases filled with law books enclosed in glass against the wall. The floor inside the office was exactly like the floor on the outside - wood.

There was no way to sneak into Dallas Knapp's office. Every step clambered loudly and echoed back in all directions. You could hear any visitor coming long before they hit the landing at the top of the stairs. There were no other noises to compete with the unmistakable sound of footsteps climbing up the second floor. It was otherwise a very sterile quiet environment.

Dallas Knapp sat behind a large wooden desk. His office had one dominant color – brown. There were no carpets or rugs or drapes to soften the noise of footsteps climbing the stairs and entering his office. No way to know in advance that might be coming, only that someone was coming. But, his visitor needed no introduction.

"Howdy, Will."

They quickly shook hands. Both men gripped the other's hand firmly and shared mutual smiles.

"I know you're here to settle up on that real estate matter we talked about, but, first, let me ask you, what is that you've got there in your shirt pocket? It looks like a long nail." Dallas gave a bewildered look and shook his head.

"That's exactly what it is, and I call it my Hooch Tester." He removed it from his breast level shirt pocket and showed a long nail held between his palms.

"And what do you do with a "Hooch Tester?" He cocked his head dubiously.

"I use it." He smiled. "Whenever anybody offers me a drink, that's when I use it. I dip the nail right into the drink, all the way to the bottom, and then I take it out and sniff it. If I smell even the slightest trace of alcohol, I pass it back and say no thanks. I don't drink any kind of whiskey, and I can always smell it." He put extra emphasis on the "always."

"Oh. A hooch tester. Hmmm? I guess I'll have to get one of those, Will." They both laughed. Grandfather Knapp did take a drink every so often, but he was careful about it. They both knew he'd never use it if he did get one. The legendary cowboy winked at him and they started doing their business together.

Dad would always say there were just too many lawyers for such a small town in Kansas, and the economy wasn't good in that area. Dad was a victim of his own choices, and a poor example for me to follow in terms of my own success. I looked up to him for doing things perfectly, but I guess he wasn't very good at choosing to do the things that could have made him successful or wealthy.

Maybe bad decisions and bad choices were just something in the air, lingering latently from the past, long before Dad was born there.

2

COFFEYVILLE IS FAMOUS for a very explosive historic event back in 1892. A group of brothers, Bob Dalton, Emmott Dalton, and Gratton Dalton had gained a reputation for themselves as horse stealers and train robbers. Frank Dalton was also a brother, but he was honest, and stayed away from his lawbreaking kin. Sadly, he was killed in the line of duty working as a US Deputy Marshall in 1890.

With their brother dead, the remaining Dalton brothers wanted to do something greater than the famous Jesse James had ever done, and maybe get revenge for their brother's death. So, they tried something never done before - to rob two banks at the same time – the First National Bank and the CM Condon and Capital Bank. Both banks were across the street from each other in downtown Coffeyville, Kansas.

They failed miserably. Two Dalton brothers were killed and several others on both sides, robbers and city defenders, lost their lives that day. It put Coffeyville on the map for the wrong reason. It's really a quiet peaceful town now. Downtown they have a Dalton Museum for visitors to absorb the brutality of the Dalton brothers in their heyday, and to commemorate the citizen heroes who were killed trying to stop them.

Sometimes the local townspeople have a re-enactment of that historic day, dress up like cowboys and shoot each other up with blanks. Then everyone claps and they all have a celebration.

Dad liked using big words. I knew he had to be really smart because he always used big words. "Very definitely." "Virtually impossible." "Non-denominational". "Unequivocal," "Mellifluous." I don't think there was anything he didn't know. And if there was such a thing, he would stop and go look it up. To me he was a genius and a hero.

I saw him many times reach quickly for the dictionary, read pointedly for a few seconds, smile, and return the book to its place on the bookshelf. He always smiled when he had a complete understanding about the subject of the moment. Sometimes he would then give me a wink to let me know he was totally satisfied with the outcome and there was nothing more to search. Other times he would laugh quietly to himself as if there was some secret joke and only he was in on it.

He once sat me down and read out of the first few pages of the dictionary. "If the word you are looking for is not in it's proper place in alphabetical order, then it is not in the book at all."

Isn't that wonderful?" he asked me gleefully. Then he laughed to himself. "Not in the book at all."

3

I WAS BORN knee high to a grass hopper in Coffeyville, Kansas, on June 26, 1949. Mom survived many weeks of over 100 degree days with no air conditioning to deliver me in the new hospital there. Soon after I came into the world Dad returned to the service.

We lived in Norfolk, Virginia, in an apartment on the second floor, and he was in the Navy. Once when I was two years old. I was really sick with a fever. I was crying my head off as you would expect a baby to do if he felt that bad.

"Please be quiet there." Mom tried to hold me still. "Shut up, quiet there, little fella. Stephen. Please." Dad became quite sharp.

But, I did not respond to his appeals. I guess he was used to always getting his way when he commanded someone. He had his uniform on and had just gotten off a ship. I was not in the Navy and must have been feeling too awful to cooperate.

Whap! He hit me hard across the face with the palm of his hand.

It happened that Mom gave me some aspirin just a few minutes before Dad hit me. His hand print turned bright red on my face and I continued to cry even louder than before.

"Oh. Charles. Look at him!" Mom was mortified. The thought of me walking around the rest of my life with his hand print etched in crimson on my face was horrifying to her.

Dad smiled. "He'll be all right." He lit a cigarette. Mom shielded me in case he did it again and they walked to their car.

"You'll be all right, Stephen. You be strong now. Everything will be just fabulous, just wait and see." Mom comforted me.

It cleared up later that day, but he never hit me in the face again.

That Christmas we went to Indianapolis to see my mom's parents, one set of my grandparents, Charles Robert and Sophy Bispham Weiss. My grandfather, GrandDaddy Weiss, was a mechanical engineer for Link-Belt and he designed linkage for large earth moving machines. He was a successful man and provided well for Grandmother Weiss. He had a big heart and a great sense of humor. Everybody called him "Skeet." He liked telling jokes and making people laugh.

"Let's see what I have in my pocket," he'd say. "Well, looky there," and he'd give me a red Life Saver out of the roll he had half-way already used up. He seemed to never run out of Life Savers. I thought he had a big box of them stashed away somewhere. "How about a red one, or do you like the green ones? Stick out your tongue. Isn't that just grand?"

My grandmother spent most of her time gathering in social circles and doing whatever social ladies do. She played bridge and canasta, and probably other games, too. She was always at home when I saw her. Sitting and looking charming and graceful. She was small and petite like my mom. She had a permanent smile on her face. Mom told me once that grandmother Weiss had three miscarriages when she was young. She figured they were probably boys and she was just too small to carry them. Too bad, really. I could have had three more uncles to play with growing up.

She kept the housekeeper, Amanda, pretty busy cleaning, washing and cooking. Ding-a ling. Ding-a ling. Ding – a – ling. Whenever she needed something she would ring a little glass bell, always close by on the nearest table, and Amanda would rush to politely ask what she wanted her to do next. "Amanda, could you adjust the blinds, please, it's a little bright in here presently. Amanda, I think we'll have lemonade in the living room. Would anyone like anything else? Bring some potato chips in a basket, also. Thank you."

My grandmother Weiss was proper, dignified, composed. Never in a rush. It was always quiet and calm in their house. Except for their dog, Vicky. A black cocker spaniel. She always wanted me to pet her. Vicky often broke the silence when she barked when someone came to the door.

Amanda came to work every day on a bus. All the housekeepers would get off just before 5 PM and stand by the bus stop two houses down from my grandparent's house.

I never saw them talk to each other or laugh, but maybe they did that when they got in their seats.

Both Mom and Dad smoked cigarettes. Camels, unfiltered. Dad had a Zippo lighter that he carried in his pocket. Mom used a lighter on a table, or matches from the kitchen. There were ashtrays in every room.

Dad would take his cigarette and tap it against his lighter. I guess he thought it burned better if it was firm on the tip, or maybe he just liked smashing his cigarettes. Mom had been taught in college how to smoke properly. She made smoking an art form. Her hands moved like a ballerina, and both lighting and smoking it and blowing out the smoke were full of elegant maneuvers to look like movie stars and sophisticated adults.

A few days after Christmas GrandDaddy Weiss was holding me on his lap one evening and talking to me while making funny faces. "Well, well. Aren't you something?" His eyes were wide open and he grinned from ear to ear. "You'll be a big boy some day, won't you? And you'll be so smart, just like your father." He bounced me up and down on his leg as he chanted, "Boom a laddy. Boom a laddy. Boom. Boom Boom."

Suddenly, I slipped out of his hands. My face hit the brass wastebasket by his chair as I fell. The top edge of the round wastebasket caught my left eye. Blood gushed everywhere.

After I landed on the white thick carpet there was a brief moment of complete silence. Then Oooooooh! Aaaaaaaaaaaay! I cried louder than I ever had before in my whole life. It wasn't even a cry. It was more like a terrifying scream of unbelievable pain. Mom, Granny, Dad and GrandDaddy were petrified.

Dad took charge. "Oh, my God! He's bleeding. Oh, you poor fella. Get the car! We're taking him to the hospital. Let's go, let's go everybody. Quick! It's OK honey, you're going to be OK." GrandDaddy felt awful about it. It showed in his crushed look of helplessness. I continued to scream, Mom held me close to her breast, soaking her dress in blood. Everyone else sat silently as my Dad drove, praying for the best, too afraid to even consider the worst. If I was going to grow up to be the All American boy, I would need both my eyes.

My left eye was so swollen for five days I couldn't see out of it, but the swelling subsided and the eye healed back to normal. The black and blue colors which imbued the left half my face faded and disappeared. I could see just fine once I was able to open my eye.

All that remained was a deep gash just to the outside of my left eye. I missed being permanently blind in one eye by a half an inch. My head sustained a violent shock, but everyone was only worried about my eye.

My head had taken two big wallops before my third birthday. I'll never know if anything inside my head had been affected. All the damage appeared on the outside of my head and that's what got all the attention. Only many years later would I learn that head trauma may lead to MS and that physical and cognitive symptoms of MS could develop early in childhood. All my future problems may have started with brain damage stemming from one or both of these instances.

We returned to our apartment in Norfolk, Virginia, and then moved to a house in Virginia Beach. By then I was as good as ever. Fit and as fiddle, Mom would say. She never played any fiddle so I don't know how she knew to say that, but it seemed I was OK. The house we moved into was only about a block from the beach. Mom and I took walks up and down the beach. I played at the edge of the water and the ocean waves would chase me back toward the dry sand.

"Mom, look. What is that? Why is he so funny looking?" I was always curious and asking questions, but Mom didn't always answer back. I think it was because she didn't know. Dad always answered me.

I had found a small crab. She called them fiddlers. We watched it crawl back into its hole as the water rushed to fill the hole. We watched the sea gulls and I would pick up feathers that they had left behind. We could see the big ships come in and go out all day long from the harbor.

"Come here, Stephen. I've got to get your feet clean." When we walked home from the beach and I would have tar on the bottoms of my feet. Her solution was to put turpentine on a rag and rub each foot with the rag. It smelled terrible, but it worked. I got a turpentine foot rubdown every time we went to the beach.

One day I woke from my nap and couldn't find Mom in the house. I yelled over and over but there was no mom. No Mom? I thought maybe she took a walk on the beach by herself so I went to look for her.

I wandered off by myself and started looking for Mom. She had been next door, and became frantic when I wasn't there. After searching the house and the neighborhood Mom called the police. I was found an hour later by a life guard on the beach. The problem had been that I was lost. I had no idea which way to go to get back to the opening where I entered the beach. At the age of four it was apparent I had a poor sense of direction, which would cause me major problems throughout all my life. This was just the first indication. Mom was too scared and upset to worry about that. She was just glad I was found.

"What were you trying to do, give me gray hair early? Never, never, never do that again." She had that serious look on her. She lectured me about the dangers I had luckily escaped, and how I might not be so lucky the next time. People drowned every day she told me. I couldn't be too careful. I would never grow up to be the All American boy if I let the ocean take me away forever. That made sense.

Early in my toilet training I got scared sitting on the stool to do number two. Number one was no problem because I was just tall enough so that I could do it like Dad did. But, I cried doing number two because it made me afraid. It was a big seat and there was a big hole in the middle of it. My balance wasn't that great. There was nothing to hold on to and I was afraid I was going to fall in.

Mom said to try sitting backwards facing the wall. I had to take my shoes off and my jeans off and my underpants, but when I sat on the stool I felt safe. There was a pipe I could hold on to next to the flusher handle. On some toilets I could put my elbows on the big lid or reach out a hold on to a towel hanging on the wall. I liked it that way better. I like going "backwards."

For the next two years or so when I said I needed to go "backwards" Mom knew what I was talking about. When it finally got to be too much trouble to take my shoes and my pants off every time I had to go I started doing it the regular way. By the time we left Virginia Beach I wasn't scared to sit the other way like Mom and Dad did.

After Dad's time in the Navy was over we headed back to Kansas. I sat in the back seat most of the time, but sometimes I would stand on the seat and lean forward, and I would be right between Mom and Dad. They always sat in the front seat and I always sat in the back seat of Dad's car.

I was standing up on the seat and leaning forward and I heard Dad talk about finding a nice home.

"What do you mean? We don't have a home anymore? Where are we going to live? Where will I put my toys? Where will I sleep? This is terrible. What's wrong with our old house? I liked it just fine."

"We're moving to Kansas, Stephen. Your Daddy is going work there. We'll live in Coffeyville where you were born."

"Where?"

"We don't know yet, Darling. But, don't worry. We'll just have to wait and see what Daddy finds for us. He's going to find something very nice. Just wait and see. He's not going to leave us homeless."

Mom always ended those kinds of conversations with a smile. A big one where she raised her shoulders and grinned for ear to ear.

It was a long hot trip half way across the country and I worried as I sat in the back seat. Homeless was not something I had ever heard of, but it didn't sound like something I would like. Her smile lingered as if to add more reassurance to her comments.

I was very curious about where we were going to live when we got there and I was upset there was not already a house waiting for us to move into.

"How could that be, Mom?"

"How come we don't have a house? We've always had a home and a place to sleep. Am I going to have to sleep on the ground?"

She said warmly, "No, Stephen. We'll stay at your grandfather Knapp's house for a few days."

"Do they have a beach there?"

"No. Not in Kansas. Sorry, dear."

We stayed for a few weeks with my other set of grandparents, Dallas William and Mildred Smith Knapp who resided in Coffeyville, Kansas. Coffeyville was the town where I was born and it became my home until I was raised.

4

I GREW UP hearing Coffeyville being referred to as a "dinner-bucket" town. No frills. No ostentatious displays. No conspicuous consumption. Everybody lived a quiet non-descript, conservative lifestyle. Everybody knew everybody, and there were no secrets. And no place to hide if you really embarrassed yourself, so most people avoided attention all together.

There were, on the high side, about 12,000 folks who lived there. The year was 1953. It was a friendly, safe small Midwestern town, and a great place to grow up in. No one locked their house or their car. In fact, Mom and Dad left the keys in their car. It was very easy to get around. From one side of town to the other took less than ten minutes driving time. But, there's no reason to go that far. Across the tracks was "Colored Town."

We never went there until I was much older.

Coffeyville was not a very big town. Half the streets were named after trees like Pecan, or Walnut or Elm Street. The other half were numbers like First Street, Fourth Street and on up to about Fifteenth or Sixteenth Street. Then on the west side are some streets with other kinds of names. They all ran pretty straight. Far on the east side of town was the Virdigris River.

Past the Virdigris River was South Coffeyville, but it was in Oklahoma, so that really didn't count. Besides, people over there talked funny. They all had southern accents and said words like "ya'll." Mom and Dad never used that word. They just said "you."

Coffeyville still had cable cars for public transportation which ran down the important parts of town. I liked to hear the electricity cackle over the cars as they moved along the streets. They disappeared not long after we moved there.

Dad found a house. Across the street from it was a wheat field. I've never lived close to a wheat field before, but I could sure smell it. I sniffed the air. There was a distinguishable odor of rich warm earth, dust and live plants. It was spring in Kansas and the stalks were just starting to turn golden on top. They reminded me of the tassels that hung from the big chandelier in Grandfather Knapp's dining room over the table where we ate, only there they were somewhat of a reddish color.

In the evening I watched the sunset. It was hot and humid and sweat rolled down my forehead stinging my eyes. The sky was orange and the sun was a big giant ball slowly sinking under the ground beyond the wheat field. There was just enough wind to make the wheat sway as it rustled, flowing like waves in the ocean. It reminded me of where we used to live in Virginia Beach. But, there was no beach, no sand, or no ocean where we lived in Kansas. It was all different.

I liked watching lightning bugs flash their glowing tails as they disappeared and reappeared over the field. I heard crickets singing loudly to each other. Locust's music filled the air from the neighbor's trees, and pesky mosquitoes tried to drive me inside.

They liked to bite me, and when they did, I got big red swollen sores for a few hours that were hard to not scratch, and it always made it itch worse when I did.

It didn't take me long to become an expert on all the bugs around there. I liked bugs. I liked lady bugs and June bugs. I liked grasshoppers and crickets. I liked rolly polly bugs that hid under rocks with the white grub worms. I liked butterflies, too. All kinds of colors. Little tiny yellow ones and black ones. And big ones that had orange wings. This turned out to be a whole new world for me.

"Pssst. Stephen. Come here. Dad whispered and wiggled his cupped his hand telling me to come with him. We're going out." Mom was asleep.

A few minutes later I got my first real hair cut at a barber shop. Dad's barber shop. I was almost four and I had never had one before. Until then people who didn't know me thought I was a girl. Dad snuck me there to avoid an argument with mom. I never heard them argue. They agreed on most things. I never heard what Mom said about it, but I had a burr for the next ten years or so. Never needed a comb once.

Not long after we moved here the locals decided to start a country club and golf course. Coffeyville did not have one that was private and there was enough interest to make it become a reality. There was a municipal golf course on Big Hill just out north of town, but it wasn't a nice course. Its nick name was "the Goat-ranch."

We joined as charter members of the new country club which was the beginning step in a lifelong enjoyment of the game for me, plus a whole lot more.

One Saturday afternoon all the new members came out to work on the new course which was about to be built. There were kids, adults, dogs – it was a real gathering. We had to remove the rocks and throw them into one of several pick-up trucks which would haul the rocks away. This was the first step before they planted grass, built the nine greens and nine tees. The following year it would be completed - Coffeyville Country Club. They talked about where the club house would go and how the golf course would be designed. Where the 9th green would be. Where the first tee would go. No body knew yet but everybody had an opinion about it.

I had to do something to help out. "Ouch! These rocks are too tough to pull out for me. I'm just gonna do the little ones. They don't hurt me. Hey, Daddy. I'm just going to do the little ones."

"Just do what you can." Dad smiled and lit a cigarette.

"Hey, look! A turtle. A turtle, Mom. Look. A terrapin slowly ambled past the crowd of workers paying no attention to them and what they were doing. "Look Dad, a turtle."

"Oh, isn't he funny?" Mom wasn't really watching it, and we certainly did not share the same degree of fascination.

"Hey, there's another one." I ran to inspect the strange red and yellow markings on his shell.

"What are those things called?" I was looking at a brown little creature with spikes on its back and its head.

Pete Stover offered, "We call those horny toads." Someone said, "You'll see a lot of 'em around here. Don't worry, they won't hurt you. And they're more scared of you."

It dashed off and disappeared before I could get close to it. Cecil Jones laughed.

I watched Dad play golf once when I was five, just after the new course was open. He played with three other men. They all had their clubs and their bags sat on pull carts. I tried to pull the cart myself but it was hard at first. And heavy. But, I liked being outside. When it got really hot, I didn't mind that either. I liked being with Dad, and he was willing to let me go along as long as I followed the rules:

No talking when someone is hitting.

No walking when someone is hitting. Stand very still.

No yelling, ever.

No getting in front of someone who is hitting.

Never step on the line of someone's putt.

Never step right by the hole on the green.

Never pull the cart onto the green. Go around it.

Don't scrape your feet on the green. Pick your feet up.

Always be courteous and polite.

Sounds like a lot of rules, but I had to learn them or I couldn't go. So, the choice was easy.

I called some of the men Dad played with "Mr.", like Mr. Wall, Mr. Strausburger, Mr. Pratt. And then there were some doctors that played with my Dad. Dr. Coyle, Dr. Grigsby. It was a chance for me to get to know all my Dad's friends. And learn a very wonderful game with men who taught me a lot about how to act on the course just by watching them. They were true gentlemen, good sports, loved the game, were very competitive, and funny at times.

"Nice shot, Charley."

"Not too bad, there, Ken."

"Ooooh, Nice one, Jack."

"Dandy, John."

"Well, it not that good, but it's handy."

"You're away."

"No, go ahead, I'm not ready."

"Beauty, Chas."

"OK, Podsy. Get it close, I'm in my pocket."

"Nice putt, Alice. Need a few more Wheaties on that one!"

And, they liked to gamble among each other. But, only in small amounts. Two dollar Nassua was the usual bet. Two dollars for who ever wins the front and two more for who ever wins the back, and two dollars more for whoever wins the whole round. Unless someone presses, which is like starting a new bet, you win or lose up to six dollars for the day. It was a team game so they decided who were partners by throwing all four balls into the air and the two closest were partners. Simple. No argument. Always fair. Everybody had a handicap but they were honest about that. They always played together. So there was no way to fudge a score. They all played by the rules of golf and they had a deep and abiding respect for the game and its integrity. They were all great character models. At least, when they were on the golf course.

5

MY BEDROOM WAS plain. The walls were blue, the ceiling was white. The floor was wood. I had a small bed that stood on four wooden legs. I had a three drawer dresser, but the drawers were much bigger than my clothes. My shorts, my jeans, my underwear, and my sweater just about filled one drawer, so I had two empty drawers with nothing to put in them. I had a closet with four shirts. Two white ones and two blue ones all on fancy little blue and white hangers.

Mom believed all clothes should be able to "mix and match." As long as I only had blue and white, there was never a problem with clashing colors.

Mom took me all the way to Kansas City once to buy clothes. We went to a place in a hotel room where piles of different samples were laid on big flat tables. She called the brand Best & Company. We spent about three hours there.

Two weeks later my new clothes arrived. Two white shirts, and one navy blue shirt and a pair of navy blue shorts. Life was simple in those days.

Mom and Dad had a party one night. They had dinner and drinks and coffee and lots of other stuff. I slept through it. But, early next morning I got up and they were still asleep. Dirty dishes and glasses and cups covered the dining room table.

I'd never tasted coffee before. Mom always said it was too hot. It sure wasn't hot then. So, I took a big black swig of it out of a half empty cup.

"Ughhhhhhhhhhhhhhhhhhhhhhh. Yuck!" I almost threw up. I thought the taste was the most horrible liquid I had ever had in my mouth. That's it! That's the last time ever. I'll never drink coffee again.

It was not until college when I needed a way to stay up late that I ever tried coffee again. And I flavored it with tons of milk and sugar so it had no chance of resembling the cold brackish coffee taste that still lingered in my taste bud memory files.

At age four I started rocking my bed at night. My legs felt funny, weird, and I had to move them or something to go to sleep. I couldn't just lie in bed and feel my legs feel funny so I got up on my knees like I was praying. Then I leaned over so my head was on the sheet and my knees were close to my chin. I pushed back and forth with my legs moving me forward and backwards. Sometimes I would make up songs in my mind and I would rock my body to the rhythm of the songs I heard in my head.

Screech. Screech. Screech. Screech.......

"Stephen? Are you all right? What's that noise? What are you doing?" Mom heard the bed posts scratching against the wood floor and she came into me bedroom to check on it.

"I'm OK. I'm just not tired yet. Just rocking myself to sleep, mom." She looked at me on my knees in my praying position, but she didn't say anything about it. She just smiled.

"OK. Good night, Little lovebug. Don't let the bed bugs bite," she said softly and smiled again. For years I would rock my bed assuming the same position night after night.

"Nighty, night." I resumed my rocking until much later when I fell asleep.

"Whoa. What's this?" In the morning I opened my eyes to a strange sight. The room moved. No. Somebody moved my bed with me in it while I was sleeping. I got out of bed wondering why my bed had moved all the way across the room to the other side. What was…..Oh, the rocking. It was the rocking.

Every night after that I got in bed on one side of the room and in the morning it was on the other side of the room. It was the rocking. I rocked my bed across the room because I couldn't take the feelings in my legs. I couldn't lay still and go to sleep. I had to rock and exhaust myself until slumber greeted my sagging eyes and fatiguing body.

Occasionally I would rub the pillow case with my forehead hard enough a mark, like a blister, would show where I had touched the fabric over and over.

6

KINDERGARTEN. SCHOOL. I went to a brand new school just built called Edgewood Elementary School. It was 1955. It would be my school for the next seven years, kindergarten through sixth grade. The new school was six blocks from my house and it was right across the street from the smelter, a paint factory for Sherwin-Williams.

The smelter made a really disgusting smell like rotten eggs, sulfur, and once in a while the wind would blow so that no one could help but breathe it. I liked the smelter because it had a big whistle that was so loud people could hear it all over town. It blew at 12 o'clock noon and at 5 o'clock. I never needed to know what time it was. I just listened for the whistle.

Mom bought a rug for me to take a nap on at school. Everybody in kindergarten had one. I never slept on it, I couldn't sleep on the floor like that, but I did rock on it sometimes. Some kids gave me some really strange looks. I just shrugged my shoulders. I didn't care. I liked to do it.

The rug was not as smooth as my pillow and I started rubbing a sore on my forehead. In a few days it showed and Mom asked where it came from. "What's that mark on your forehead? Come here. Let me look at that."

"Oh, nothing. I did it at school. During our nap time, you know. I was just rocking. You know, rocking."

"Oh." She knew what I meant. She just shook her head.

In school I found another way to do something for the funny feeling in my legs. I put my feet apart and my knees banged against each other, back and forth, sort of like the Roaring Twenties dancers. This motion was soothing so I did it underneath my table, or my desk. I did it the whole time I was at school. I did it at home. I did it in Dad's car. I became a sitting knee-banger. It became a habit and it felt good.

I had an idea once to give Mom a funny Christmas present. Mom was good at wrapping packages so when she wasn't looking I wrapped one. Later I gave it to Dad and told him to keep it until we went to Indianapolis and then we could put it under the tree and gave to her then.

When the holidays rolled around I reminded Dad to bring my present in his suitcase to give to mom. He nodded.

After all the other presents were opened, Dad produced the small package. "Here, Betty, Stephen gave you this." My grandparents looked on wondering what their grandson had given his mother.

She pulled of the ribbon and unwrapped the paper. Then she peered into the box, and shook it. Then she turned it upside down.

"It's empty!"

"Hah. Hah. Hah."

I thought that was extremely funny. An empty box.

No one laughed.

Dad and my grandmother exchanged looks of disbelief.

"Stephen. Is there another present, as well?"

"No, Mom. Just the one for a joke"

"Well. You should have packed two. It's OK to play a joke, but you should have made it right with a second one. That would have been the proper thing to do."

"OK. Next time. Sorry."

I heard them talking about me later, but they were whispering so I couldn't pick it up.

I was fascinated by watching the squirrels run and jump in the front yard of my grandparent's big white house. The trees were huge and the squirrels seemed to love to play going up and down the many branches that grew up from their large trunks. I decided I had to catch a squirrel.

I figured if I was quick enough I could hide behind a trunk and run around to the other side before the squirrel knew I was there. I crouched behind the tree waiting to put my plan into action.

In one smooth movement I stepped around the tree, stuck out my hand and grabbed the squirrel's tail. It was bushy and course, not soft. The squirrel froze. I froze. We stared for just a moment into each other's eyes.

In what probably was less than a second it occurred to me I had no plan for what to do next. I had done what I set out to do. I caught it. I had no clue what I should do after that, so I let it go. Not surprisingly it disappeared quickly. Dad said I was lucky I didn't get bit later when I bragged about my "big catch". I never tried that again. But, I still enjoyed watching them.

Mrs. Miller went to the office one day and asked the operator for CL1-5422. The operator made the connection. Rrrrring. Rrrrring. Our black phone at home on the wall was ringing.

"Mrs. Knapp. Is this Mrs. Knapp? Hi. It's Mrs. Miller, Stephen's kindergarten teacher. I am concerned about Stephen. I think he needs his adenoids checked. He sits in class with his mouth open. Yeah, for a long time every day. He holds his head still like he is in a trance, his legs wobble back and forth, and he stares into outer space with his mouth wide open. I think you should have him checked. I just wanted you to know what I thought.

Oh, yeah, he's doing great in school. He's a bright boy. All his grades are good. He's not having any problems, but I think you should have him checked. Bye, now."

What in the world is she talking about? There's nothing wrong with me. I didn't say anything. I pretended like I didn't hear her and I didn't know what was going on.

Mom followed through. Dr. Martin checked my adenoids, my tonsils, my throat, nose, ears, eyes, everything. Even my blood and my urine. He said I was normal.

Oh, yeah. That's what you think. I didn't say that, but I thought it. Funny thing was I was hoping he didn't find anything, but I figured there had to be something there. Maybe he just missed it.

The chicken pox was going around the school and I got it. So did most of my friends. Lucky me. For three days I had to stay at home. I wore my pajamas all day long and never took them off. I could run all over the house, but I couldn't go to school. I couldn't go outside. I was like prisoner in my own house. Just me and Mom and the old RCA radio.

We listened to Arthur Godfrey and The Breakfast Club with Don McNeil, and a lot of other people I didn't know, but once in a while they played a song I liked. I turned up the volume when Ernie Ford sang "16 Tons." Mom brought me coloring books but I got bored and went to sleep. "Can I go to school today? Tomorrow, maybe?"

"Oh, Mom this is absolutely awful." I did get better reading, but it was a lonely time.

Later that same year I got the measles. Mom caught them from me so we both had a good being sick together time. I hated not being in school because everyone else was there but me. I could only listen to a radio so long before it started making funny noises and then I turned it off. The next week three other kids in my class got it. Mom said measles was just one of those things going all around town.

Mom invited some of my friends to my birthday party. The first thing we did was go to the Tackett movie theater and saw "The Wizard of Oz." I really liked it but I didn't know why only the first part of it was black and white.

Coffeyville had three movie theaters, the Fox, the Tackett and the Midland. All of them had wads of gum stuck underneath the seats. Thousands of them.

7

WHEN I WAS six, Dad bought me a set of junior golf clubs -a 3-wood, a 5-iron, a 7-iron, a 9-iron and a putter. They came in a bag I could carry with a shoulder strap. Dad gave me a few of his old balls and I was all fixed up. I started playing a few times and I started to caddy for him on weekends. Actually, I pulled his cart. I was interested and wanted to play.

Smack! "Beauty, Mom. Nice shot. Right down the middle. Watch me now." We played together, just Mom and me on my first round. Thank goodness it was just the two of us.

Whiff! I missed it. Whiff. Missed again. Click. I moved the ball forward a few feet. It was a lot harder than it looked, but I could do it better. I would do it better. I couldn't make it go like Dad did.

Something was definitely wrong? Very definitely.

After three holes I started crying. I exploded. "Dang it.! I can't do it." I lost my temper. I hated playing. I hated doing badly. I couldn't make it go like Dad could. I wanted to do it better than he could.

"Stephen. Just slow down. Don't look up." She always said that as if it was the panacea for all of golf's ills.

"Thanks, Mom." I was steaming mad. I kicked the ground.

We finally finished nine holes. My score was 103. I counted every shot and wrote it down on my scorecard. Mom's score was 65. We were both pretty bad. But, I knew I could do better and in time I would.

I learned it was important to keep the ball clean while playing, especially on the greens. The men carried towels on their bags to clean off the balls. Sometimes big chunks of mud would stick to one side and there was no way the ball was going to roll straight with all that mud on it.

For many years the golf course at Coffeyville Country Club was run on a very small budget. There were no watered fairways. There were no sand traps, no cart paths, no manicured golf course. No flowers. Just nine tees, nine fairways and nine greens. The greens were small, but well kept.

The fairways were Bermuda grass, but spotty. There were bare patches and plenty of crab grass, clover and dandelion weeds. Sometimes the ground was so dry it shrunk with cracks bigger than my finger. I would see dust curl up into a tiny tornado and spin around a while. Then it would disappear as fast as it came up. In the summer the course baked in the sun. So did I.

Shorty Watts was the greens keeper and he was a crew of one. He did everything he could and he worked seven days a week from before sunrise to sunset. He drove a four gang mower. He mowed the greens with a push mower. He changed the cups. He mowed the tees and set the tee markers, the white ones for men's and red ones for the lady's. He was good at it, and he worked very hard. He even put water and soap into the ball washers.

Twice a year he would aerate the greens by punching holes in them, covering them with sand and fertilizer and overseeding them with rye until the bent grass came back. The greens looked dead in the winter, but they were beautiful and green in the summer.

Shorty was always nice to me. He'd usually tip his hat towards me, or just nod and smile. His skin was dark from sun burn and his face was rough. He had a red scarf he wore around his neck. He always wore an old blue cap. His teeth were stained from years of chewing tobacco, and he was missing two teeth.

"Go ahead, there." He motioned for me to walk in front of him and he slowed his mower down to a stop and turned it off so it didn't make any noise. He was always polite, always friendly.

Shorty would water the greens by hooking up a long hose to a large sprinkler and, one green at a time, he would water them down. A few times a year he would fertilize the greens to keep them healthy. Dad said the greens were more expensive than anything else on the course.

Caddying was hard work, and even though Dad paid me five dollars, he let me take a few breaks. Like when two holes were side by side each other, I could just bring a driver, and a putter and leave all the rest of the clubs to get when we passed the golf bag going the other way to the next hole. Sometimes this meant I didn't have the towel when Dad got to the green to clean it off. So, I would just lick the ball off and rub it against my pants. I watched the men do it, so I figured it was OK.

No telling how much fertilizer I put into my mouth. But, I continued this practice of occasionally licking my golf ball for my own playing through college, not realizing the potential dangers. There were a mixture of chemicals to help the healthy grass grow and other agents to kill the weeds. It was highly poisonous and could have made me sick or worse. Sometimes it actually tasted good, but not all fertilizers tasted the same. I didn't know it was poison. I just knew a clean ball was better than a dirty one. I didn't want anything to make me miss a putt if I could help it.

Coffeyville was located on the map in the southeast corner of Kansas, 3 miles of Oklahoma and 50 miles from Missouri. It was in the Midwest part of the United States, and the Midwest was plagued with Dutch Elm's disease, which killed thousands of beautiful elm trees. In Coffeyville Elm trees formed a canopy over 4th street for many blocks through the town before the Dutch Elm disease made the city look naked with all the dead trees that had to be cut and removed.

Following other cities with the same tree disease, Coffeyville flew planes dumping large quantities of DDT into the air to try and stop the disease from getting worse. Anyone who was outside like I was all the time got a few snorts of DDT in their lungs here and there, maybe a lot of it on some days. So, besides the fertilizer I picked up on the golf course, I had mixed it with DDT in my lungs. Both substances passed deadly particles to my bloodstream and into my brain. But, I was so healthy who would have ever suspected anything. I'll never know if I incurred any damage from ingesting DDT.

8

I GRADUATED TO first grade, but so did everybody else in my class. It wasn't hard. Miss Harris was my first grade teacher. She was tall, pretty and had black hair. She wore bright red lipstick. She must have liked red on her, but not on me.

Paul Kiser and I were outside swinging at recess. The brisk autumn wind blew hard from my right to my left and Paul was swinging next to me on my right. Paul decided to bail out of his swing. He landed awkwardly on the ground and fell forward and caught himself. Maybe he told me he was going to do that, but the wind was so strong I wouldn't have heard him anyway.

Whap! I felt metal crack against my left forehead. The wind wildly blew Paul's swing sideways, past me and snapped back to hit me hard just above my left eye. The bolt that links the chain to the seat smacked me solidly, and I bailed out not really knowing how bad it was. I just knew I'd been hit by a swing.

The south-westerly gale was so strong it was hard to walk straight and I had to lean into the wind or let it push me over. Blood ran down my face, across my shirt, and down my pants. By the time I walked through the classroom door I was a bloody mess.

Before I could tell her what happened Ms. Harris looked up at me and fainted.

Mr. Butterfield, the principal, called my Mom and she took me to the hospital. It was the same hospital where I was born, just only one block down the street from my school. They gave me four stitches in the emergency room.

The stitches were very close to the scar I got when I fell on the brass waste basket.

Mom looked at me one day and frowned. She told me "We need to put more meat on those bones, Stevo. I'm going to start filling you up. I want you to clean your plate every meal. Those poor children in China are starving, you know. Here, this will give you plenty of vim and vigor." She gave me her usual wide smile.

That's just what I needed, more vim and vigor, whatever that was.

She gave me a large helping of cottage cheese on a plate with some Ritz crackers topped with slices of Velveeta cheese. She had covered the cottage cheese with sugar to make it taste better because she knew I didn't like cottage cheese. It tasted OK with the sugar so I ate it. That became an every day snack, and I usually got some more for dinner.

Mom and Dad came home with new puppy, a Great Dane that they named Dana. I liked Dana and I learned how to house train a dog so she wouldn't make a mess on the floor.

Dana had to have her ears cropped, which Dad said would make her ears stick straight up after it was done. She had bandages wrapped around her ears for a while, but when the vet took them off, sure enough, her ears always pointed toward the sky.

One day Dad left early to go to work, and Mom went shopping. I went to open the door to go to school and Dana suddenly pushed her way past me through the door. I tried to get her back inside but she was too big and didn't always listen to me. I had to go to school or I would be tardy which I never wanted to be. Only the bad kids ever were tardy and I didn't want to be one of them.

"Stay, Dana. Stay," I said. "Please," I pleaded with her. She just wagged her tail and hung out her tongue and pranced her way following me to school. It was five blocks to school and I didn't know how to ride a bike like the bigger kids so I had to walk. "Stay. Dana." No luck.

By the time I got to school lots of kids were playing outside waiting for the bell. When they saw her they came up and tried to pet her.

"Here, boy. That's a good dog. Wow. That's a big dog. What's his name?"

"It's a she, not a he. Her name is Dana." By now there were a lot of kids crowded around us. I guess they'd never seen a Great Dane before, especially right by the school. Dana weighed 60 pounds and was bigger than some of the kids. The bell rang.

RRRRRRRRRRRRRRRRing.

Everybody went inside and she followed the crowd. Inside the hallway kids started screaming. I called for her, but, it was too loud in the hallway. It was very crowded, it was loud and I'm sure Dana was scared. I lost sight of her. I was scared for her, and for me.

"Is this your dog, Stephen?" Mr. Butterfield had grabbed Dana's collar.

"Yes, Sir. She's mine. She snuck out of the house and followed me to school. I couldn't make her go back. She's too big for me."

"Let's go into the office and call your home. Tell the operator to connect me with Stephen Knapp's number, Della. What's your number, there, Stephen?"

Dana sat quietly, and yawned while Mr. Butterfield kept her still.

"CL1-2472," I told him. Mom had made me memorize it just in case. All he really needed was the last four numbers, 2472, everyone in Coffeyville only had four numbers, but I knew CL stood for Clinton and I wanted to show him I knew the whole number.

"Hello, operator. 2472 please......."

He talked to Mom and I went to my home room. Somehow he got Dana in his car and took her to my house. When I got home I expected Dad to be furious with me, but he wasn't.

"Well now. I hear you had some real excitement today, didn't you? Just don't let that happen again, son. Be more careful next time."

"OK. Sorry."

That was it. I was expecting him to get really mad, but he didn't. I guess I was just lucky that time.

A year later I still didn't have much meat on my bones and I was the second shortest kid in my class. But, worse than that, I had to go to the dentist. Dr. Shanahan was nice and so was his wife. They worked together. He gave me X-rays and a few days later he called and told Mom I had 9 cavities. He took two days to do everything, one day for my right side and one day for my left side. After both sides were finished I had nine fillings. Nine mercury fillings. All that sugar, mostly from on top of the cottage cheese plus missing some brushings showed me something. So, bad things could happen to me. I thought I was bullet proof like Superman. Especially with that powdered tooth paste that tasted so good, I thought I'd always stay far away from Mr. Tooth Decay, but I was wrong.

It was Christmas Day and Dad surprised us with a real Deusey. After we had opened all the presents there was knock at the door.

"Who's there?" Mom said. Dana barked like crazy. It was someone she didn't recognize.

Dad said, "Why, it's Joe Claus. Hi, Joe! Merry Christmas! Whatcha got there, Joe?" Dad had a way of asking questions when I know he already knew the answer. I recognized Joe when he walked in because he worked at a store downtown, but he was wearing a red cap with jingle bells on it.

I wasn't expecting him to bring in a big RCA TV set, but he did.

"Where do you want it to go Mr. Knapp?"

"There." Dad pointed to a wall in the family room. "It'll fit absolutely perfectly right there."

Dad asked him questions about his family and was he going to be able to spend time with them.

"Oh, yeah. Just two more stops and my Christmas begins. Got a big roasted ham waitin' for me at home. I can almost smell it now. Heh, heh."

He hooked up the TV, gave us a quick 1-2-3 about how to turn it on and find all three channels – ABC, NBC, and CBS. And he showed us what to do when the picture flips and rolls. He made it do that and then he twisted the knob to make it stop. It was our first black and white TV ever. I was excited to watch it, but at the moment it was just showing a picture of an Indian, so we had to keep turning it on and off to see if anything else was there. He showed Dad how to correct the picture if it starting flipping. That would come in handy later on.

"Ya'all have a nice Christmas, now. Bye."

"Bye, Joe," we waved to him.

"Thanks Joe and Merry Christmas to you and your family."

It was cold outside. The winter weather had made everything turn brown and all the trees, the maples, the oaks, and the elms, had lost all their leaves. The wind made it even colder as the sun hid behind dark, gray clouds. I would shiver if I stayed outside very long, even wearing my gloves, my stocking cap and my winter coat. And my nose would sting, too.

We had a nice Christmas tree with lights and tinsel. Santa Claus brought me presents and Joe Claus brought a TV. It didn't get any better than that.

A few weeks later everybody in the neighborhood started taking down the holiday decorations and put their old dried out Christmas tree on the edge of the yard so it would get picked up. A couple of the older kids, Stuart Martin and Dick Wade, decided to collect all the trees from around the neighborhood and build a fort. That took up a whole Saturday afternoon, but it was great fun. I had a lot of fun living around a bunch of creative kids. We played together a lot. It was a great neighborhood to grow up in.

9

WE WERE DOING an art project one day in class at Edgewood. We were coloring a drawing of a country scene. I had a cow, a horse, a barn, a bird, clouds, sky and the sun in my picture. And some green grass. It wasn't very special, actually sort of ordinary, I guess. I wasn't a great artist. I felt fine at the time, but that wasn't going to last long.

"All right, now. Put your crayons and your poster away. We will be walking to Mrs. Wilson's class." My teacher was making us move to another classroom. I had all my crayons in the box, but I didn't close the lid. All the second graders took music in Mrs. Wilson's room.

We were walking single file and suddenly my head went into a spin. I felt kind of dizzy and like someone was trying to pull me into the darkness. I fought to not be pulled away. I was no longer in the room with the students. My world was fuzzy and I was being forced to do something strange….. and then it was over. I fell and my crayons went all over the floor. A lot of them broke, which I hated because I couldn't color with a little bitty short crayon.

"Stephen. What's the matter with you? Watch where you're going, boy. Clean up this mess and hurry up about it." Mrs. Wilson didn't understand what had just happened. She didn't ask, either. She thought I was just fooling around. I wasn't.

I just about passed out. Maybe I almost died. I don't know. Everything went blank for a few seconds. I didn't know where I was or what was happening to me. Then it was too late. I felt stupid picking up my broken crayons, but I didn't say anything. What could I? No one would understand, so I kept quiet about it. It was weird, but it never happened again.

I got an invitation to a birthday party at the skating rink. Just about half of everybody in my class got one. It was my friend Bill Beine's birthday. He was going to be 7. His birthday was June 1st, mine was June 26th. He always had his birthday before I had mine, every year.

He was one of my friends and he lived right behind my house. His Dad was a doctor. He had an older sister, Stephanie, and a younger brother, Bob. Bob was born with a limp and couldn't run very fast. But, we all played together and it wasn't talked about. Bob didn't skate at all that day.

The party was fun except I fell a lot. I usually had good balance. I ran fast, I jumped, I dribbled a basket ball, I could hit a tennis ball, I could catch a foot ball, I could hit a golf ball really far, I could punt a football, I swam, I dove off the diving board, I could do a lot of things pretty well. But, in skating I had a problem with balance. I was always leaning too far forwards or too far backwards. I couldn't get the hang of it.

I had the same problem in the winter trying to skate on ice. No balance. There was a lake in the middle of Coffeyville Country Club and I borrowed Mom's skates one time and went with some friends. It didn't make sense. I could ride my bike with no hands. I even got in trouble once doing that when Mr. Butterfield caught me on the way to school. I had balance with everything else, but not roller skates. I couldn't figure it out.

The next summer we went to Iowa to visit my Dad's college room-mate when they were at Kansas University in Lawrence, Kansas. He lived in a Spencer but his family stayed in a summer house on Lake Okoboji and he had a boat. The water was so clear I could see the bottom like it was right next to my hand, but the water was really way over my head.

Dad taught me how to water ski. I wasn't very good at it, either. It was fun to go so fast, but I never felt comfortable on skis. I was afraid to lean back.

ZZZZZZZT. ZZZZZZZT. The boat's engine roared louder as it went faster. I felt the power surge as I lifted out of the water, and then on top of the water, skipping the surface like a flat rock.

"Hey, look at me. I'm doing it. Whoops!" Splash! "Dang it!" I said to myself.

Just as I started making a smooth wake I fell forward, and let go of the rope. My life jacket kept me floating and they came around to give me another chance to get up. After five more chances I nearly had it down, the standing up part anyway, but my legs felt like they were shaking and they were never holding me up very well. I felt shaky the whole time on the skis. I now know these were tremors caused from MS, but I had no idea then why I was shaking. I wasn't nervous. I just accepted it.

But, this was all new, so what was it supposed to feel like? I didn't know. I just felt like I wasn't going to be very good at it. For some reason, I just knew water skiing was not my sport. Living in Kansas, that was not going to be a big problem anyway.

We stopped the skiing that day when Dad had an accident. He got the rope twisted up and it went through his legs and burned the inside of both his thighs. When he wore shorts his rope burns showed for most of the summer. It must have really hurt but he never said anything.

In third grade Mom decided it was time for me to get piano lessons. She had taken lessons for years as a child and she played beautifully, although not very often. And when she did, she usually had to have the sheet music in front of her or she couldn't play but just a few songs. I thought that was weird. Seemed to me once you learned it, you could play it.

My first day with Mrs. Winkle was hard for both of us. She kept trying to get me to put my fingers in position with them straight up and down like letter L's. I couldn't hold them like that and I kept flattening them out which made her mad after a while. She kept reminding me, and several times she grabbed my fingers and forced them into the proper position.

"Do it like this. Hold your hands in this position. No. Not like that, like this. Here."

She bent my fingers.

My knuckles didn't want to move like she wanted. It hurt me the way she put them on the key board. It was ridiculous to think I could actually move them when I was in that much pain.. Mom said this would be fun. Hardly.

Then we started the first book of songs. C – D - E….. C – D - E.

That was it? That's not a song at all. But I played it. C – D – E. over and over. Yuk.

After four lessons I had mastered one simple song, "The Songbird," and she put me into a recital. I had to get all dressed up. Mom oozed all over with pride as I played it with no mistakes, but it was too easy. Everybody clapped, even people I didn't know.

In the car leaving I told mom, "Mom, I don't wanna play that stuff. I wanna play real songs. Mrs. Winkle doesn't know any real songs. I don't want to go anymore."

"OK. Dear." She smiled. "You may wish some day you stayed with it, but I'm not going to make you do it."

And that was that.

I still wanted to play so I got my little record player that plays 45's and 33's, and put it on top of our grand piano. I liked the song "Exodus" by Ferrante and Teicher, so I played it on the record player and listened. I hit a few keys, searching for a couple of notes that I heard in the song. I listened to the record more, and went back to hitting piano notes. Back and forth, back and forth, until I had the song figured out. Not the complicated fancy stuff, just the simple melody. I played a few basic chords that made the song sound right. Later Dad taught me about minor and major chords that night, and said I sounded great.

"Mom, listen to this," and I played what I had taught myself with Dad's help.

"Oh, honey, that's fabulous." That was her favorite word, "fabulous." She used it for everything, so I wasn't sure it was that great but it sounded OK to me.

"I couldn't do that. How did you do that? Oh, you have your father's ear. He can do that."

I knew what she meant. I had heard him. He played "Tea for Two" every time he sat down at the piano. Then he pecked out "Stardust," but he didn't have that one "quite under his belt yet," so he told me. We didn't have sheet music for "Tea for Two" or "Stardust". He just knew how they went by heart.

Once when he played Dad started thinking of the war and he started reflecting on the past few years before I was born.

There were two stories I never forgot although I heard them for the first time and he never repeated them. I always gave him 100% attention when he told me stories. I was always amazed and felt small and dumb by his intelligence, his broad experience, his insights and I was usually caught off guard by his dry humor. There were no humorous moments on this occasion.

"We were on the surface,' he told me, "and I was on watch. I was at the bow, the far end you know, furthest from the hatch. I spotted two enemy planes and we had to go under immediately. I yelled, "Let's go! Everybody down! Planes! Three o'clock"

"What's that mean, Dad? Three o'clock?"

He said, "The sky watch is like the face of a clock. 12 o'clock was due north. 3 o'clock was due east." He moved his flat hand to his right for three o'clock.

"Then 6 o'clock is due south, right?" I pointed my finger toward the bottom of my other palm.

He nodded.

"OK. I got it."

He continued.

"There were, oh, I guess about 10 men on deck and they all rushed to get below. We had to get off the deck quickly or we were not going to make it. The sub had already started to submerge, and waves were coming over the deck. A big wave hit me and threw me over the edge. My boot caught on a post that held up a short fence -like structure. The last man, Bill Robinson, going down the hatch just happened to be looking in the right direction to see my boot. I was fighting seawater in my mouth, and I was in the ocean except for my leg. He went back up the ladder, ran and pulled me out, and helped carry me to the hatch. Just as we got inside, the door slammed shut. The door was sealed. And immediately thereafter we were under water. And we were safe. I coughed up water for the next 30 minutes, or so, but, other than that, I was all right."

"I spent that night thinking about what I'd been through. I decided there must be a God, and He had a plan for me and I still had work to do to finish His plan. For the life of me, I didn't know what that plan was. But, surely the sequence of events that saved my life could only have happened if some Greater Power had been on board with us. I swore that night I would never take the Lord's name in vain again for the rest of my life."

I didn't know what to say at first. We just looked at each other. There wasn't really anything I could say. But, I know my heart was beating hard.

I finally said, "Well, I guess if that guy Robinson hadn't saved you, I wouldn't be here. So, I'm glad that he did."

"Affirmative."

Dad usually did not talk about his war times in the Navy. He would make a frowning face which told me he wanted to talk about other things. If I asked him a question he would say "Affirmative." And nod his head. Or, "Negative." And his head and face would be still without any expression.

But, this time he continued with a second story. "Stephen, would you like me to tell you a story about another incident when I was on the Hake submarine?"

"Affirmative, Dad." We both smiled.

"We were experiencing depth charges," he told me, "exploding in the water close to us. We were under the water, but they had radar and could estimate fairly closely just where we were located. All they had to do was set the charge to go off at a certain depth and BOOM! BOOM! BOOM!" He made very loud noises, hitting his hand on the kitchen counter, trying to make sure I knew it was a very loud sound.

"If they guessed right we would have been blown to pieces and I wouldn't be here talking to you." He smiled again. Dad had an expression on his face that he was almost cocky about what he was talking about. I had seen that expression often when he knew he was right about something..

"Fortunately, for both of us, they missed."

"All the men were very scared. All our electrical systems were cut off so they could not find us on their screen. Or, at least, it made it more difficult. We sat there in the dark listening to the deafening sounds of the depth charges exploding. We prayed for our lives. Praying we would get out alive. Praying we would see our wives and families again soon."

"When one hit particularly close by, the sub shook and rocked back and forth. Anything that wasn't securely tied down flew and scattered around the ship." He flipped his hands outward as he talked about what a mess it was, 'But nobody cared about the mess. They were thinking about their families. They wanted to come home when the war was over."

"We aimed, torpedoed and sunk three Japanese ships during my time there. I am not proud of that, not at all. But it was necessary. We had our orders." His face was solemn, and his forehead wrinkled. "There is no glory in killing. None, whatsoever. I can tell you that. Very definitely, none."

I've never seen him look more serious. It must have deeply affected him to shoot down people. His whole body slunk almost in shame. It was a very personal experience for him. And for me, too, just to hear about it.

He always talked because it was related to something else. There was a greater message that I was supposed to get. That's why he told me that story. I was supposed to appreciate that we were a family. There was a story on the news about some racial killings in Alabama and that worked its way around to fit into Dad's story. We were supposed to appreciate that we lived in a safe place and we were alive. And free.

"Thanks for telling me that one, Dad." I idolized my Dad. Whatever he said I took in and committed it to memory. He was always right. He was the perfect father. To my young and very biased mind he could do no wrong.

10

DAD BOUGHT MOM a new 1957 Ford Fairlane convertible. Charcoal gray with a white top. I thought it was the prettiest car in the whole town. It got so much attention Dad was invited to drive it in the city Christmas parade and also for the high school home coming night at the half time. We took lots of Sunday afternoon drives into the country with the top down.

A new car turned heads in Coffeyville. And, of course, we had to pass through town to get out of town, so we didn't exactly sneak away without being seen.

The car reminded me of Dad. When he went to work he always wore a suit, a charcoal gray suit, and a white cotton dress shirt, long sleeves with a button down collar. And a striped tie, his favorite was navy and burgundy. The tie didn't exactly go with the car, but the suit and the shirt sure did.

Mom liked to sing a song by Benny Goodman about Flat Foot Floogey with the Floy Floy. I never had any idea what that was all about but she always smiled after she sang it. Then she'd sort of pull in her shoulders and smile at me again. She liked to listen to Patti Page sing, a famous female recording singer. Mom told she got that name because Page Milk Company, here in Coffeyville, helped get her started making records.

I drank Page milk every day. Lots of it. Gallons, half gallons, quarts, pints - you name it. Page Milk also made the cottage cheese that helped me get nine cavities. It was the sugar, of course, but I ate it all together.

Mom managed to live without ever getting upset about anything. She had an inner strength that she just accepted things even when she could have really sounded off. She never argued. She never got mad. When things seemed to go wrong, she just smiled and raised her shoulders. She never seemed to have any real big problems she had to face. Life was always calm. Or, at least, it looked that way.

She had her opinions. Things were "good, fair to middling, fabulous, or no good at all." A lot of things were the "finest in the United States." She had a real sense of judging quality. She liked to use superlatives. Nothing was average. It was the "worst", "most horrible" item imaginable, or it was the "most elegant" item in the world she had ever seen.

One day, we became a two-car family. We had two cars in our driveway. Most people only had one car. We only had one garage, but we had two cars. Dad had a white Chevy station wagon, and Mom had the convertible. We were living "high on the hog" as Dad would say.

In the summer we went to Leland, Michigan, in the new car. After driving a few days we were in Milwaukee, and we got on a ferry boat to cross Big Blue, or Lake Michigan. I guess Dad missed being on a ship and that was as close he could find. I never saw any boats in Kansas. No oceans, no big lakes, no submarines. Kansas was flat and very solid ground. There were creeks and little ponds, but not like this.

It was dark. I watched the water get pushed away by the front of the ferry boat. There was white foam crawling up at the top of the wake, I just stared at the water for a long time.

I wondered what it would be like to jump in. What would happen? I thought about it. I pictured myself in the water, disappearing under the dark water and the white-capped waves pouring over me. Mom and Dad would not be too happy. I could die. A lot of people might scream or be mad at me. I didn't know. They may have thought I was weird or crazy. I sat there still and quiet listening to the motor grunt and groan, and the water splash.

I didn't do it. It wasn't like I was afraid. It wasn't like I was nervous. I was trying to think what it would feel like, and I wasn't sure.

I never said anything about it to Mom or Dad. It was one of those moments I just kept everything inside.

They looked over and smiled at me and I smile back. "Everything's OK. How much longer?"

"We're traveling at about 10 knots." Dad changed his voice and sounded like he was back in the Navy. "I'd estimate maybe another hour, more or less."

Dad was definitely talking Navy talk. He lit a Camel cigarette, and took a big puff and let it out.

"What are knots? I thought that was what I made to tie my shoes."

He smiled. "Knots are a measure of speed when you are on the water. It's the speed of one nautical mile and takes into account the curvature of the earth."

"Oh."

I didn't exactly get that, actually, it was way over my head, but I was too tired anyway. "Is there somewhere I can lie down? I'm so sleepy."

We had a nice time in Leland, Michigan. Dad and I played golf once, just the two of us. I wanted to beat him, but he was still way too good for me. Some day that would change. I was driven to beat him. It was always in the back of my mind.

On the drive back home we stopped in St. Louis. Dad found a little restaurant for lunch that was real fancy. All the waiters wore black coats and ties.

There was a man, also in a black coat, playing the violin, going table to table taking requests. I never heard any of the songs he played at the other tables. When he got to our table Dad asked me what I wanted to hear. It was July.

"I'll pick Jingle Bells." Mom laughed. Dad nodded his approval and he played it, perfectly.

It was boring sitting in the back seat all alone. I turned around and began counting the white stripe that divided the highway into lanes. By the time we got home I had counted up to about 100,000 of them.

I told Dad my accomplishment. He said, "In my book that's a lot of stripes."

11

IN FEBRUARY, DAD announced he had made plans for a trip to Monterey, Mexico, and we would spend two weeks with his old college room-mate, John, Maggie, his wife and their daughter, Jenny, who was seven.

We had to talk to my teacher about taking me out of school.

"Here's what I want you to do, Stephen." My third grade teacher made it fun for me.

"Every day you are gone, I want you to write down in a diary about everything you did that day. A draw pictures of what you saw. When you get back, you can read it and show to the class and then we will all learn some things about Mexico by sharing your trip."

"OK. Sounds fine with me. I'll do it"

Mom and I bought a Big Chief notebook and a sketch pad, crayons, pencils and erasures just for the trip. I was going to make a really good report.

I had to get a bunch of shots at the doctor and have my picture taken for a passport. I guess that was normal stuff. Mom and Dad did it, too.

We flew to San Antonio to catch the plane to Mexico, but it was too foggy and so we spent the night there.

It was so hard to see one time John was afraid the cab driver was going to wreck his cab.

"Alto! Alto!"

I quickly figured that was Spanish for "Stop."

I looked at my window early the next morning and saw the Alamo across the street from out hotel. The sun was bright and the air was fresh and crisp. I sketched a picture of the Alamo. That was my first drawing.

After breakfast we walked around and there was a big limestone fire place in the lobby with a baby alligator swimming in a cut-out brick area just to the right of the fireplace. When we walked outside I noticed a beautiful letter "A" in an unusual script inlaid in the cement as we walked in by the front door which was the first letter in the hotel's name – Ancira. I wanted to walk around more but Mom said it was time to catch the plane.

Monterrey, Mexico, was so different that I had never seen anything to compare with it. The money was different. The language was different and I didn't understand any of it. Their dollar was called a peso. Twelve pesos equaled one US dollar. Little boys and girls with no shoes and dirty faces ran through the streets. The girls were selling tiny boxes of Chiclets gum, and the boys were shining shoes for a penny. I had never seen anything like that in Kansas.

"Chicle, senor?"

"No, gracias." Dad taught me how to say that on the plane, just in case I actually talked to someone, and I did.

I played golf two times with Dad and John, and I had to have a caddie. It was the rules there. I only had six clubs, a 3-wood, 3-5-7-9 irons and a putter. And a little red carry bag. My caddie was at least

60 years old. I felt like I should be caddying for him. He was older than Dad. It was strange just to have a caddie. That was a first. I guess there's a first for everything.

Dad said the next day we would ride burrows through the country. It was fun. We had a guide so we were safe, even though the roads were rough. They didn't walk very fast. And it kind of bumpy, but it was fun.

I saw my first waterfall. It was beautiful to see so much water going straight down and splashing into the lake at the bottom. It looked a lot like the hair on the tails of the donkeys, gracefully falling.

We stopped at the home of a large family, living in the middle of nowhere in a one room house out in the country just off a dirt road.

"Alto!" The guide gave directions to the driver.

We met a man, the father of the family, who made baskets from straw and Dad bought one for each of us and some straw hats. It was hot, dirty and flies were everywhere. I felt sorry all the boys and girls who lived there, I counted eight children. I didn't even see a bathroom. I was ready to go home after that.

Mom and Dad had gotten over from what they called "Montezuma's Revenge." We stayed in our hotel room and they used the bathroom a lot. I drew pictures of Monterrey and wrote a lot on my Big Chief tablet that day about everything I had seen.

We had fresh fruit every day, which was great. The Mexican food was OK, but I liked my lunches and dinners at home better. At home I ate hot dogs, and peanut butter sandwiches, or egg salad sandwiches, and macaroni and cheese. Fried chicken I missed, terribly. Mexico didn't seem to have any of my favorite foods. They had tons of fruit and we had fresh orange juice every breakfast, but no Sugar Pops or Rice Crispies.

Dad helped me write a seven page report when we returned and I read it to my class. Every so often, I would stop and show them something like a basket, or a coin, or gum, or my drawings, or the noise – making clackety clack castanets we brought back with us. Everybody clapped when I finished my report. Then it was back to the usual routine.

Leland, Michigan is a special place to everyone in my family on Mom's side. GrandDaddy and Granny Weiss were always there for the summer. It was Mom's second home. She spent her summers growing up here with her parents and Aunt Hebby, her sister.

Mom had asthma during her younger years and GrandDaddy Weiss bought a place in New Jersey as a summer vacation spot which was supposed to be a better location for her health, but it wasn't. So, he sold it and bought a lake front cottage on the beach in Leland, Michigan, which agreed with her much better as it was cooler and had a lower humidity.

Aunt Hebby was always fun to be with. She liked to play games with GrandDaddy and she taught me how to play backgammon, and cribbage and dominoes. They were hard to learn at first, but I got better the more I played them.

Dad and GrandDaddy played cribbage and kept score on a special cribbage board with holes and pegs. For hours they would play. But, I learned how to play just watching them.

Leland was a sleepy small fishing village on Lake Michigan. Most people only stayed there for the summer because it got so cold in the winter and it snowed so much. All of GrandDaddy and Granny's friends, and Aunt Hebby's friends were summer residents only. They lived in Indianapolis or Chicago or some other place the rest of the year.

When we arrived at the cottage I ran through it, hardly noticing the inside, and stopped to take in the magnificent view. Beyond the two-story white cottage was two levels of grass as the terrain sloped toward the water. There were three wooden steps which lead to the beach. Towering white birch trees and pine trees lined both sides of the lawn, but all trees stopped at the beach, and there was about seventy feet of pure clean sand before it met with the waves of Lake Michigan. There were little wet rocks on the edge of the beach which rolled in and out with the water. Sea gulls flew overhead and there were two islands, North and South Manitou, visible several miles off the shore. To me this was, and still is, paradise. It was a view that has not changed for me in over 50 years.

Just outside the cottage on the lake side in the upper section of the yard stood a white brick pedestal. There was a brass sun dial on top of it. It told the time and the month according to where its shadow marked the time line. GrandDaddy taught me how to read it, and he compared it to his watch. The sun dial and his wrist watch always matched. I was amazed how it could do that. Of course, it had to be sunny, but it usually was.

I ran along the beach and threw rocks into the water, and watched the seagulls. They were majestic in the way they would swoop into the water trying to catch a fish, and fly back up in one smooth motion. Other times I watched them seem to hang completely still in the air as they flew into the wind. We didn't have seagulls in Kansas. They were pretty tame, but I never got real close to one. They would always fly away.

Sea gull feathers fascinated me. There were always some on the beach. I picked up their fallen white and gray feathers with white stems that were like plastic straws and felt them. They weighed absolutely nothing.

Mom and Dad liked to sit on the front lawn, a level above where the beach started, and talk. The cottage sat on ground much higher than the beach and sloped down toward the sand, and ran even lower gradually to the water. It was always a relaxing spot to be in overlooking the water.

Hebby taught me how to skip the rocks so they would sort of bounce on the water's surface. I learned that flat rocks skipped much better than round ones. And small flat rocks went better than big heavy flat rocks. With a good rock, I could make it skip ten or more times before it sank. If the water was real calm, when there weren't any waves at all, sometimes a lot more times than that.

Dad took me out to the golf course. It was only nine holes, just like in Kansas. The last hole was weird because you couldn't see the green. It was a short hole, but it went straight up a hill so steep it was too much for me to climb pulling his cart. You could just see the top of the flag. I you looked through a contraption similar to a periscope on a submarine, you could see if everyone in front was off the green so the next group could hit safely. Dad hit one and it disappeared in the sky.

"I think I hit a good one, Stephen." We looked everywhere when we got to the top of the hill. We found it in the hole when we got to the top where the green was. A month later we received a case of Wheaties for his hole-in-one.

My uncle, Gary, was always fun to be around. He was tall, handsome, sunburned with white sun-bleached hair and had a good sense of humor.

"Hey, everyone. Let's go take a boat ride." Uncle Gary had a small boat which he kept on Lake Lelanau. That was a small lake just beside Lake Michigan and it flowed into the big lake down this little canal which connected them. There were hardly any waves on the little lake. He had more planned than just riding the boat.

"Hey. Want to catch some fish for dinner tonight? Here, put a worm on your hook, Steve. Let me show you how." I had never fished before. What an adventure!

Uncle Gary had bought worms and had fishing poles ready in his boat for all of us. He handed me the shortest one.

"Wow. I've never done this before. I don't know how."

"Watch me, Steve. Don't let them bite you. Just kidding. Worms won't bite you."

I knew that much. I'd seen worms in Kansas hiding under rocks.

"Look. They are still alive!" The worm in my finger wiggled.

Gary was much taller than Dad, and he was tan so he must have been outside quite a bit. He had blonde hair like me, but his skin was red. His shoulders were wide and he looked very strong. I liked his smile. He seemed to be happy we were there.

He was tough, too. I watched him take a swim in Lake Michigan every morning we were there. The water was always very cold, some days colder than others, but he went in any way. He even took soap with him and took a bath in the lake. I'd never seen anybody do that before.

"OK. Watch this closely now." He stuck the hook through the worm three times. Then he threw the line into the water.

"Now you wait until you feel a bite and then you pull up like this." He showed me how to lift up and pull the string to make the fish come to you. Then he handed me the pole.

"Stephen, you have a fishing pole, a line and bait. You are ready to be an official fisherman."

We puttered around the lake fishing and riding the boat. We waved at people in other boats who were waving at us. This was a really friendly place. I never even got a nibble, so I was not lucky that day, but it was fun. Dad caught two little ones, but he threw them back.

He said, "You don't keep those kind, they are too small. Let them live so they can get big someday. We only keep the big ones." And, we didn't catch any big ones. Well, so much for catching our dinner. " Maybe next time."

"All right, let's go try the big lake. Lake Michigan!" Gary told us we may not catch anything there, either, if they just weren't biting, but we would see a difference in the water. Man was he right about that.

It had been so calm on Lake Lelanau the boat was riding like it was barely moving. On Lake Michigan we rocked up and down as he hit ever wave. The seats were wood and they were hard. I kept feeling my butt hurt on each wave and I didn't like it, but I didn't say anything. It was nice for him to take the time to give us a ride.

We finally stopped and hooked our worms again. But, again, we weren't lucky.

Gary and Dad talked but I couldn't hear what they were saying. The roar of the boat's engine and the rocking of the waves against the boat made it hard to hear anything else.

Mom didn't say much. She just smiled at me and was hoping I was having a good time.

We ate white fish for dinner that night at the Bluebird. It's Mom's favorite place to eat in Leland. That night after dinner I watched Dad and GrandDaddy play cribbage until I got tired and went to bed. My rear end was still a little sore from the boat ride.

The next day I met Nick and John. They were our summer neighbors who stayed two cottages down. John was my age and Nick was one year younger. John was taller than I was, Nick was a little shorter. They looked pretty normal.

"Hi," we all said to each other when Aunt Hebby introduced us.

"How would you boys like to see some big sand dunes?" We all said sure. She drove us to a place called Sleeping Bear Dunes, the world's largest sand dunes, and along the way she told us an old Indian legend about how it got its name.

"There were three bears," Aunt Hebby began, looking at me off and on to see if I was following her story," a mother and two cubs. They were on the Wisconsin shore and they were starving, so the mother told them they should all swim to Michigan. First, one cub got too tired and drowned. Then getting close, but still not to shore yet, the second cub died the same way. He was just too exhausted to go any further. The mother bear became very, very sad. Suddenly, two islands, North Manitou and South Manitou, rose from the bottom of Lake Michigan to mark the places where her two cubs had died. Years later, when the mother bear died all alone, there grew a big sand dune in the shape of a bear, standing high enough to watch over the two islands, which marked where the mother was and could forever watch and mourn her lost children."

Hebby was almost in tears the way she told it, and I was a little shook up, myself.

As she drove up to let us off she said, "See up there," and she pointed to the top of the first hill. "When you get up there, especially since it's a beautiful clear day today, you will see the two islands in the story."

"I'll come back and pick you up here in, say, three hours. See you then. Have fun."

"Bye. Thanks."

She drove off.

John says, "This will be outstanding." He mentioned he had done it before and he wanted to take the lead.

"Go ahead, John. Show us the way." There were the biggest hills of sand that I have ever seen in front of us. We started climbing to explore the first big hill.

"We'll go straight up here." He pointed to the highest point.

"It's going to get hot." He took off his shirt and tied it around his waist. Nick and I did the same. I figured he knew what he was doing so I just went along following his guidance.

The sand had millions of footprints from people who had been there before us. The sand was soft and deep and had no firm ground below it. It was hard to walk uphill in the sand and I could feel my legs getting tired. But, I could talk and do that, too. We were just climbing and talking. I didn't want them to think I couldn't do it. We stopped and turned around. John stretched out his arm and pointed his finger.

"OK," said John. "Look. There they are. There is South Manitou and North Manitou, just like your aunt said."

It was beautiful standing there. The sky was pale blue, the lake was dark blue, with little white caps lazily popping up and disappearing. The two islands stuck out dramatically as the only things in the water.

"Now that is Fox Island," and he proudly pointed far to the right of where we were looking. "And those are freighters over there. Nick and I listened as we watched him point in the direction of the two ships. I could tell he liked to be one the one who knew everything, but that was all right. It was fun being there and I was learning things I didn't know.

"Let's go this way." He charged toward another higher dune. Nick and I followed close behind him. I was starting to get thirsty. They probably were, too, but we didn't talk about it.

"I came this way the last time I was here and when you get to the top you can see for miles and miles down the beach." Never had he sounded more confident to me. I became envious of his knowledge and his self assurance.

"You sure?" Nick questioned.

"Yeah. Sure. 100% sure"

When we got to the top all we could see was sand in every direction.

"What is this, my big brother?" He said sarcastically as he opened his both arms and palms and raised them over his shoulders. Beads of sweat dripped down Nick's face in disgust.

"Slight miscalculation. Let's go this way." And we were off again climbing to our right and up some more. Now I was really getting thirsty, and tired. Worry started trickling into my mind.

"Uh. Something is not right here," John said as we reached the top. "All we can see is more sand. That's not what I'm supposed to see."

"Funny thing. The millions of footprints we've been walking over have disappeared. Where'd they go?" I asked.

"We're someplace new. This is cool. Nobody's been here before." John was pleased.

"Yeah, but how do we get back? I'll bet Aunt Hebby will be looking for us."

"No problem. Let's go this way," John directed us, and we were off again. We didn't see another human being, or even a sea gull, for the next hour, and I was sure we were completely lost. No trees, no houses, no Lake Michigan. Just smooth golden sand, and then more sand, and more sand after that.

"There they are!" It was some men that looked like police but they were in some special Jeep, wearing red jackets, pointing to us and waving.

"We're here. We're here!" We waved back. They found us. We rode with them, gulping water all the way down.

Hebby was waiting as we drove up to her car. She was not happy to see us.

"Thanks for finding them, gentlemen," she smiled. "They won't do that again. You can count on that. Right boys?" Nick glared at John. No one answered her.

"Sure thing, Mrs. Richardson. Happens all the time."

As they drove off she said, "What happened to you guys?" Her angry eyes demanded an answer.

"Oh, nothing. We were just exploring," John said.

John and Nick's Mom and Dad were there, too. I went back with Aunt Hebby.

We said good bye to them. "It's very simple," I told her. "We got lost. It all looked the same. Sand here. Sand there. Sand, sand, everywhere. I was scared."

Once again, not having a good sense of direction made me get in trouble and feel stupid.

At breakfast everybody was planning their morning. Granny was going to sit on the porch. Grand-Daddy was going to play golf with Dad. Aunt Hebby and Mom were going to go play tennis.

Just as I was wondering what I was going to do John knocked on the door.

"Hey. Nick and I are going to go over to the cliffs and look around. Want to go along?"

"Think you can do that without getting lost?" Dad said, winking at me.

John quickly responded, "Oh, yeah. Sure. It's easy there. The road is always close by. No way to get lost." He answered looking confident, almost cocky.

"Bye." Dad said. "Be careful."

"OK. Bye Mom. Bye Dad." And, we were off for another adventurous day of exploring.

The cliffs turned out to a lot of climbing just like yesterday, but not quite as steep. There were trees and tall grass and funny looking weeds. I had a good time, and we never got lost once. Not even close to lost.

I was hot and when I got back to the cottage my arms itched. I scratched them and they itched more. My legs started itching, too. My skin had red spots all over. My neck started itching.

"Hey, Mom. Look at my arms. What's going on? I'm itching like crazy."

"Uh, oh. Stephen." Mom screwed up her face like she was stumped doing a puzzle. "I think you have poison ivy. Heb, what do you think? Look at his arms."

"Oh, brother. That's it. You got it good, too. Let's go down to the Merc and see what they have for it."

The Merc was like the general store for everything. Food, beer, snacks, orange juice, vegetables, medicine. They had everything. Aunt Hebby found some pink salve and walked to the register.

"This is all they have. It'll have to do."

"OK."

This was all new to me. I had never had poison ivy before. I'd heard about it, but I've never seen it. Didn't know what to look for. Never saw it where we were in Kansas. I didn't think I had ever seen it anywhere.

We went back to the cottage and I got covered in pink salve.

"Don't touch it. Let it dry and then don't get it wet. No baths, no swimming for you, young man."

I guess Mom had some experience somewhere with pink salve and poison ivy. I sure didn't. But, I was about to learn the hard way.

Great. How lucky could I have been? What a perfect way to spend a summer. I was itching like crazy.

That night I couldn't sleep. I itched everywhere. I couldn't stand it. Every so often, I would just barely touch a place on my body somewhere that really itched. That felt good for about a second. Then it itched harder. No one could sleep feeling that.

I lay in bed listening to the waves gently roll onto the beach and barely plash against the shoreline before falling back, retreating toward the big lake. The quiet waves that usually put me to sleep now were the only thing that kept my mind from thinking about how much I itched. There weren't many places on my body where I didn't itch.

The next day I got worse. It was in my hair, in my eyes, and on my ear. It was all over my legs and my arms and my back. I had to sit inside and sweat. I couldn't move and the sweat rolled down making my skin itch worse. Mom told me if I wipe off the sweat, the poison ivy will spread. I told her it's already spread everywhere anyway.

How could it have possibly made any the difference?

I had found a totally new sense of complete misery. Everybody else was having fun but me. Nobody could have fun feeling like this. Driving for days back to Kansas wasn't any fun, either. It was a horrible thing to experience. Sitting in a hot car, sweltering heat, sweat rolling down like a shower, itching all over my body head to toe, even counting white stripes on the highway couldn't keep my mind off of how awful I felt.

The only guy feeling worse than I did was Johnny Parsons. He lived next door, and he was a few years older than I was. His father managed the Oklahoma Tire & Supply store downtown. His mother didn't work. They were always friendly neighbors to me, but I never knew them very well.

Johnny had black hair, slicked back and wore a black leather jacket. He rode a motor cycle his Dad bought him.

I didn't know any of Johnny's friends. He would take off on his bike and be gone. He rolled in late at night and the rumbling of his cycle always told me had come home. He never joined in with the other neighbor kids to play. Maybe he should have.

Just before the Fourth of July Johnny decided he would go over the border into Oklahoma. Rumor was that they had better, bigger fire crackers in Oklahoma. I guess the laws were different than in Kansas. More lenient.

He bought Black Cats in big rolls. Huge rolls. Bigger than anything I'd ever seen. Except for Cherry Bombs and M-80's they were the loudest. But, Cherry Bombs and M-80's were sold one at a time. Black Cats came 500 to a roll and they were each two inches long. A roll of Black Cats must have been three feet long just for one roll.

I don't know how many rolls Jerry bought but he had so many he couldn't carry them all, so he wrapped them around his waist. Around and around and around. He crossed back into Kansas but before he got home, which was only about two more miles, his motor cycled threw out some sparks. The sparks lit the fuse of a Black Cat fire cracker. Just one. That's all it took.

Around his waist Black Cats exploded. He wrecked his bike trying to stop and get away from the explosions, but there were too many. Pow! Pow! Pow! His skin was barbequed again and again. Each fire cracker blasted into his flesh and burned it severely.

He rolled over and over crying in pain trying to get the unlit packages off before they were ignited. He was only partially successful. He had to be taken to the hospital to the emergency room. He was there for days.

"Hey, Steve. You want to see somethin'? Come 'ere." Johnny called over to me a few days after he'd come back home.

I saw bandages around his body, his arms, his legs, and his neck. He said some even flew under his shirt and then went off under his arms. He showed me that he had more than 200 scars on all four sides of him. I remember thinking those scars would follow him closely the rest of his life.

"Where's your bike? Are you going to ride it again?"

"Yeah. In the shop now. Won't get it for a while. Needs a lot of new parts. But, it'll be like new when I get it back."

He did get it back, and it did look brand new. I don't think he bought any more Black Cats. I hope not.

I was never interested in riding a motor cycle after that. The picture in my mind of the skin around his waist, burned and singed black like roasted hot dogs left too long over a camp fire will always be a crystal clear image in my mind. I never forget pictures like that. I couldn't even if I wanted to. Some things just never go away. Some mental pictures and some memories are sometimes too hard to erase.

In early September I was walking to school and Jerry Brown pointed out some big leaves growing on a vine hanging under the branch of an oak tree. I was telling him about my bad experience. Jerry was my age and lived close to our school.

"Speaking of the devil. Look at that. That is poison ivy" he told me emphatically.

"No way, Jerry. I know what poison ivy is. I had it. I just got over it. I'm an expert on poison ivy. That must be something else. Poison ivy has a three pointed leaf. I don't see anything like that here."

Jerry was a guy who always wanted to be right, even though he wasn't most of the time. He was a nice enough guy, but I made much better grades than he did.

"Oh, yeah. It is. I'll prove it to you. Watch."

He grabbed a wad of the leaves and rubbed them on my arm. I wasn't worried because I had had a good taste of what poison ivy was all about. I remembered exactly what those five pointed star plants looked like. I had no idea what Jerry had there, but poison ivy it was not.

Next day my arm itched. By evening my left fore-arm had blown up like Popeye the Sailor. My left arm was twice the size of my right arm.

"Stephen. What have you gotten into now?" Mom had that worried look I had come to know too well. "Let's see it. What happened this time?"

I told her about what Jerry did. It looked different than when I had the poison ivy. It itched just as bad, but my arm got a whole lot bigger around.

"Let's go show this to Dr. Martin. He'll know what it is."

Mom knocked on their door. Knock. Dr. Martin lived next door so we just walked over to his house. His wife came and greeted us.

"Hi. Betty. What's up? Oh, Stephen what's with your arm, honey?" I already felt pretty dumb about it.

"Hi, Bunny. Is Hubert around? I'd like him to look at Steve's arm."

"Sure, I'll get him."

Mom told him everything. "You rubbed leaves on your arm did you? You have sensitive skin. You don't want to rub any kind of leaves on you. No matter what you want to call it. What you've got here is called "poison oak." Just put some salve on it and don't touch it or get it wet for a few days and you'll be just fine."

Boy. Did I really feel stupid then! I was right. It wasn't poison ivy. But, that didn't make it any better. And my arm itched just as bad as if it had been poison ivy.

Sometimes being right is not the most important thing.

When I reached fourth grade Dad built a basketball backboard with his new rotary table saw. He put a rim and net on it and attached it to the side of the house. I stayed outside until it was so dark you couldn't see anything just to shoot baskets. I liked golf, but I liked basketball, too.

I signed up for the fourth grade basketball team and I became a starter and the best scorer on the team. I could dribble and shoot better than anyone else. I was excellent at free throws. Our first game was against Whittier on the east side of town. All the colored people in Coffeyville lived over there. I don't know why. They were all colored boys on the Whittier team but I didn't care. I just wanted to play.

I caught the ball on the opening tip-off. I turned and raced down court as fast as I could go and made the prettiest lay-up in the world. Then the referee handed me the ball and pointed to bring it in bounds.

"No. That's wrong. I made the basket. It's their ball out." I tried to give the ball back to him.

He smiled and shook his head. "There you go, son, throw it in. The ball's in play." He blew his whistle.

I faintly heard laughing in the bleachers. I looked up at the electric score board and noticed the home team was leading 2 to 0. We were the visitors. Now the laughing made sense.

Yikes! That's when it dawned on me. I had made a basket at the wrong end. I made two points for their team. My sense of direction embarrassed me again. We lost the game by 10 points so it didn't really matter, but it was so stupid. Nobody does that. Nobody makes a basket on the wrong end.

Dad saw it. He was at the game just to watch me play.

On the way home he said, "Got a little mixed up there, aye?"

"Yeah. Dumb, wasn't it?"

"Yep. I'd say so. But, your form was perfect."

He made me feel better when he said he wanted to take me to see Wilt Chamberlain play at the University of Kansas and he did a few days later. He was a great Dad.

It was getting close to the end of school and there was a city track meet for all the schools to compete against each other. I was fast and signed up for the 50 yard dash and the high jump. I was sorry at broad jump. No idea why. There were girls that could broad jump farther than I could. High jumping was different. I could go over a bar that was about 4 feet 4 inches high and not knock it off it holder. My style of jumping was called scissor kick. I jumped up, lifted one leg over the bar and then, as that leg came down, the other leg went up and cleared the bar.

Dad showed me a picture in the paper about a guy who broke the world's record high jumping. He used a different style of jump called the California Roll. He jumped up, flattened out his body almost parallel to the ground going with both feet barely rising above the bar, then rolling the body over sideways all at the same time. I decided I should try that. Maybe I could beat everybody else at the track meet if I successfully did the California Roll.

Steve Rauch, a neighbor a few houses down, had been practicing his high jumping in his front yard. His Dad had made a high jump stand with two thin boards and a bamboo pole that could be adjusted for different heights.

I had the California Roll in my mind and I tried it once. I made it over the bamboo pole then, in the middle of the air, a terrible thought hit me. How am I supposed to land? When I scissor-kicked, which was the way I usually did it, I landed on my feet. But, I was not in the position in the air to land that way. My only option was to put out my hands to break the fall of my body as I came down.

Crack!

My left arm went limp. It felt weird. I couldn't move my left arm. I had to hold it up with my right hand. I ran home supporting my left arm with my right.

I had trouble opening the front door. I had to reposition my left arm so my right hand was free. "Mom. Look at my arm."

Cripes. My chances of winning the high jump didn't look very rosy. And I sure couldn't run a race if I had to hold my other arm.

Mom just shook her head and folded her arms. "Oh. What now, Stephen? Let's go see Dr. Martin." We walked next door to the back yard. This was getting to be a habit I didn't want.

We could smell the tantalizing, hunger creating aroma of charcoal and steaks cooking on his barbeque outside. He was standing there flipping sizzling meat with a big spatula when he saw us coming. The doctor could see right away what my problem was. It was going to take more than pink salve this time.

"Come on. Let's get you in the car. I'm going to have to set that arm right now. We'll take an X-ray Betty, but my guess is he fractured it. Not a big deal, but we need to take him in now." He was so matter of fact about it.

"But, you're having dinner. Can't it wait?" Mom was trying to be polite. He took off his apron.

"We're going now." He was firm but calm.

Right after school that day I had bought a Suicide drink and drank it on the way home before breaking my arm. It's like every kind of flavor of soda pop imaginable all mixed together.

After the X-rays they gave me something which put me to sleep in seconds. They tom to count backwards from 100, but I only made it to about 95, and I was out Then they made a cast for my left arm and put it on me. I stayed in the hospital overnight. In the middle of the night I got sick and threw up. All I could remember was seeing purple stuff all over my cast. The rest of it was a blur. The next morning it was white again. A nurse told me after breakfast I had made such a mess when I threw up, they had to change my cast, my gown, my sheets, my pillow, everything. I made it all purple.

"Sorry."

I spent the first six weeks of that summer in total misery doing almost nothing. I couldn't run, I couldn't swim. I couldn't play golf.

I couldn't ride my bicycle. And, it wasn't much fun being around my friends who were doing that stuff when I had to just watch. Wearing a cast was a very crumby way to spend a summer.

My arm would sweat and then it would itch. When I couldn't stand it any more I took a ruler and slid it between the cast and my arm. Back and forth I rubbed my itching arm.

I'm sure it looked crazy if anybody was watching, but it felt so good to me I didn't care what it looked like. It made the itching stop, at least for a while.

There were still a few weeks of summer vacation left when I got my cast off. I had to wait a few days for my arm to come back to its normal size. I thought I was deformed for life when the cast came off. Skin and bones. Most puny arm I'd ever seen. Looked nothing like my right arm. But, that didn't last long, thank goodness.

12

MOM AND DAD decided to send me to Leland by myself. I went most of the way with the Martins who had a cottage on Torch Lake which was also in Michigan. We rode a train nearly all the way. I felt right at home being with them.

I sat with their family and ate with them and talked about everything we saw out the windows. It was great to travel with neighbors I knew well. Coming back home was a different story.

Granny and GrandDaddy picked me up in Traverse City and we shopped most of the afternoon. I wanted to see the beach and skip rocks, but that had to wait until the next day. GrandDaddy gave me a gift I wasn't expecting.

"Here is something I would like you to have, Stephen." It was a box. I opened the lid and there was a watch inside. It looked old, like he had worn it for a long time before he gave it to me.

"Thank you."

I wasn't real excited about an old watch being on my wrist. I had never worn a watch before like Dad did, but an old one. I had to think about that. My friends would probably make fun of me. I didn't say that. I was just thinking it. When we got to the cottage I put the watch in my suitcase, and left it there.

A week or so later it was time for me to go home. GrandDaddy walked me to the place in the airport I got my ticket and gave them my suitcase. We waited there until I got on the plane.

I hugged him.

"Bye. Thank you for everything! I love you." I forgot to mention the watch. It was still in my suitcase.

I was on a little plane and there weren't too many people on it. But, there weren't many seats either. When I got to Chicago the plane landed and as it taxied toward the place where I get off I heard my name on the loud speaker.

"Mister Stephen Knapp. Please stay in your seat and a stewardess will be with you shortly to assist you in changing planes."

"Hello, there. Stephen? Right?" She was one of the ladies that had given me some orange juice a while ago. "I'm going to walk you over to the ticket counter to make sure you get on the right plane. Is that OK?"

"Sure. Thanks." Dad had told me I would get some help along the way when I was going home, so it didn't surprise me.

"Have you any luggage overhead? Anything you need help with?"

"No, thanks. I just have one suitcase and it's checked all the way through."

She asked me for my tickets and we walked a long way down a big room with a lot of people. It was crowded. Lots of people were talking.

We stopped. She talked to another lady for a few minutes. Then she turned around and said, "Well, there you are. You're all set. I'm going to sit with you over here. We'll be here about 20 minutes and then you will boarding the plane for St. Louis. Someone from American Airlines will meet you there and help you get on your next flight to Kansas City. How does that sound? OK?"

She waited for me to say something. It had already been figured out for me. "Sure." I said, and she smiled back.

"Just let me know if you need anything. You need to go to the restroom? It's right over there. She pointed to the signs." I looked around and I didn't see any other kids traveling alone like me. I was only ten years old. But, this was nothing unusual. People travel every day.

I got on the next plane and got my seatbelt fastened. It was a much bigger airplane than the first one. There were a lot more people on it. I watched the stewardess demonstrate all the things I was supposed to know if something went wrong. I didn't pay real close attention. I figured nothing would go wrong.

Soon after we took off my ears started feeling funny. I guess that was expected.

"Would you like some gum, honey?" A stewardess offered me a stick of Juicy Fruit.

"Thanks. Is this normal? You know. The funny feeling in my ears?"

"Oh, yes, but the gum will help and it won't last too long."

I fell asleep for most of the next part of the trip and I never chewed the gum.

When we landed in St. Louis a man from American Airlines met me walking past the plane. I was outside following the crowd who got off with me.

"Mr. Knapp? Are you Mr. Knapp?" I was getting to like being called Mr. Knapp.

"Come with me please." I followed him inside. "Let's sit over here so I can talk to you." We sat together in the crowded noisy airport in Saint Louis.

"Let me have your ticket and I'll make sure everything is OK for you to board. You just have a few minutes. Are you OK?" I nodded.

Once again everything had been planned for me. I was just along for the ride.

"Sure. Thanks."

He came back and said, "Here is your ticket, go get in that line and he steered me into a line where a lot of people were standing."

"You're checked all the way through. Have a good flight." He turned and left me standing there. I heard them call my flight number and I followed the crowd into the plane.

"What number is your seat?" A nice stewardess smiled.

"I dunno. Can you tell me?"

"Let me see. That'll be 22 A, right by the window right ahead on your right. Please take your seat. Thank you. Next."

I couldn't possibly mess up that one.

I guess they had to rush and be that way when they were busy and in a hurry. I found my seat. It wasn't long before we were in the air. No one sat beside me.

Once the plane had leveled out and we were way above the clouds a stewardess came by and stopped at my row. "Excuse me. Would you like to go up front to the cockpit and talk to the captain?" The same stewardess I saw before that looked at my ticket number smiled at me again.

"Sure!" That sounded fun. It was, too.

"Hello, there young man. I'm Captain Heller. This here is co -pilot Captain Jones. What do you think of all these dials? Have you ever flown before?"

"Well. No sir. Not by myself. Not like this. I've never seen this stuff up close."

They told me things I couldn't remember, but they were nice. Then the stewardess gave me a shiny pin shaped like an airplane with AA on it and pinned it on my shirt.

"You are an official American Airlines junior pilot now. What do you think of that, Mr. Knapp?"

"I think you are all very nice to do this for me. Thank you very much. You have so many things here, how do you remember them all?"

He laughed. "It takes a while to learn it all. You can, too, someday, if that's what you want to do.

The thought of being a pilot seemed a good idea, but I was only 10. I would have a long time to think about it.

"It sounds like a neat idea. Maybe some day I'll have the opportunity. Thanks."

There would have been no way at that time to know I would have such an opportunity offered to me, and it would be taken away from me before I could cash it in.

They served a hot dinner with fried chicken, mashed potatoes, green beans, a roll and a piece of cherry pie. Not too shabby. It was great.

"7-up, please. Thank you, ma'am." The stewardess poured a glass for me. This traveling stuff was definitely OK by me. I thought to myself being a pilot some day sounded like a pretty neat dream.

I fell asleep after reading a few pages of a magazine. I didn't wake up until we were landing. It was a bumpy landing but we made it. I had to climb down a set of steps and was pushed with a heavy gust wind once I got outside the plane's door. I held on tight to the rail.

"Mr. Knapp. Hi, there. We have a little problem." Another American Airlines man met me in Kansas City as I was walking away from the plane in line with the others in front of me who got off the plane.

I guess there is only one 10 year old kid named Stephen Knapp flying that day because they all seemed to know just who I was right away.

"There's been a change of plans. Sit down here." I did as he told me.

"Hi. I'm Dan Goldsmith and I am going to be with you for a while tonight. Don't worry. Everything is fine."

"I'm sorry but you have been bumped off the plane. You see there is a doctor's convention here and this flight has no more seats available. Your parents set you up to fly "Stand By" and that means you get on at a lower rate, but you're not guaranteed a seat."

I never heard of "Stand By" before, but I got the gist of what he told me.

"So……uh, Mr. Goldsmith. What do I do now? What happens next? How do I get home?"

"Well, son, I checked and this is the last flight going out tonight. We called your parents but they weren't home. What I am going to do is to take you home with me, feed you, and wait until the right time later on. Then we'll go down town to bus station and I will put you on a bus that will take you to your home town. That's the best I can do for you. How does that sound?"

"OK." What else could I say? He had already figured all the details out. I just went along with it. I couldn't think of anything better.

We went to his place. He cooked two frozen dinners for us and he gave me a glass of water. He lived by himself in an apartment, but it was neat and clean. He took off his coat and loosened his tie. He called somebody, probably a girl friend, and said he had a change in plans. We watched his TV for a few hours. He called my house but there was no answer. We left for the bus station.

He told me that probably no one is at my house because my parents were at the airport waiting for me there, only I wasn't on the plane and they didn't know it yet. He told me they would reach my parents and give them the details on my bus schedule and explain the reason why I was not there. He said my suitcase would be there, just not me. The suitcase was checked all the way through, and it didn't get bumped off.

I trusted Dan Goldsmith. I had to. He was kind and did everything he could do for me. He made me feel not scared. I knew I was getting extra special, out of the ordinary treatment, but, I knew everything was going to be OK. I was ready to be home. He was really nice to me. It would be over soon.

We left his apartment and drove about 20 minutes. He parked his car. We went inside and he bought a bus ticket for me.

"Coffeyville. One way. One seat." He paid some money. He put his hand on my shoulder.

"This is it pal. You've had a big day. This will be the last leg. Whew, boy," he said. He gave me a tired smile and then he yawned.

We both laughed.

I told him thank you for everything. I said if my Mom and Dad were there they would say that, too. I got on the bus and fell asleep in a few seconds after finding a seat.

I think I woke up a little bit each time the bus stopped for people to get off, or on. I was too afraid I might sleep through the place where it was my turn to get off. It wasn't until I heard "Coffeyville" that I really woke up enough to move and think about where I was. I got off the bus and ran straight into my mom's open arms. Dad was there, too. He hugged me and said, "Let's go home."

"Sounds good to me."

13

MOM RAISED ME to go to church with her at the Episcopal Church downtown. Dad never went to church. He was always reading or playing golf. She signed me up to be an alter boy which was OK. Several years later I was promoted to server and carried the cross down the aisle during the procession. I also counted all the people there to get the right amount of wafers ready for Father Basso for communion.

Church service was always peaceful and relaxing to me. I usually fell asleep during the sermon, but woke up when the organ announced that it was over and the choir started singing.

I started getting better at everything. Golf, football, swimming, basketball, school. I tried to learn a lot of big words to increase my vocabulary so Dad would be impressed.

I was always trying to get his attention I wanted his approval. I wanted him to think I was growing up. I wanted to beat him at something- some game, some puzzle, something, but he was too good at everything. I had to get older first.

I fell in love for my first time in Fifth grade. Her name was Shelley. We never kissed because I never told her my feelings. I just watched her. We talked and laughed sometimes, but I was too afraid to tell her anything. I wanted to kiss her, but I guess I wasn't ready for that yet. After a few months of heart pangs, the feelings went away. At least I found out what it felt like.

I was a fan of Howdy Doody on Saturday mornings and the Walt Disney show on Sunday evenings. I was also a regular watcher of all the western shows on TV - Gunsmoke, Roy Rogers, Rawhide, Have Gun Will Travel, Wyatt Earp, Maverick, Wagon Train, Zorro, the Lone Ranger, Bonanza, and all the others. They were all my heroes. They all lived by the same code: they never shot first, they never shot to kill, only in self-defense. They were always forgiving and willing to give the bad guy a second chance. They were kind, not cruel or nasty. They didn't cuss. They always earned people's respect in the end. They always did the right thing. And usually they ended up with a nice looking lady in the end. I wanted to be like them.

It was a windy spring day. In Kansas the southerly winds blew pretty hard when it had a mind to, sometimes so hard I could barely stand up straight. The Martins, our neighbors, hired a painter to paint their house on one of those kinds of blustery days. It was a white house, one story tall, but the paint was peeling off in a lot of places especially on the sides. It needed new paint badly.

I watched the painter brush the paint on and every so often he would have to move his ladder. When he finished for the day, he left his ladder standing for the next day. The house glistened with the nice fresh white paint. After he left, I climbed up the ladder just for curiosity. My left leg started shaking like I was trying to tap my shoe to the beat of a song except there was no song and it was doing it all by itself. I wasn't making it shake. I got down off the ladder, and the shaking stopped. I went inside. I couldn't imagine why my leg wiggled like that. I wasn't doing it. I was weird. It was MS tremors, but I did not know it.

The next morning I went outside and the Martin's house looked like pepper had been sprinkled all over it, just like when I put salt and pepper on my eggs. Dad said the wheat bugs came out of the fields at night and stuck to their house. It looked awful. The painter had to scrape it all off and paint it again. I never told anybody about my leg shaking. It was just too weird, and I didn't want to get in trouble for standing on the ladder.

The wind kicked up the dust, the pollen, the rag weed, and anything not tied down on those Kansas spring days. I stood out on my front lawn one evening as the lightening bugs started to come out and the locusts were singing all over the neighborhood.

The sun was a huge orange orb, a perfect circle, slowly descending below the horizon. The wheat field just across the road swayed in rhythm to the bursts of gusts. The soft swishing sound was as gentle as the waves lapping at night in Leland. Calming. Whispering. Endlessly flowing back and forth, their stalks not knowing or caring which way to bend. Higher up beyond the sun's light the sky turned darker in progressive patterns. The yellow turned to orange, to light blue, to dark blue and then sapphire, and darker still as the light melted into the heavens and became black.

If I had been blind at that moment, I would have known without question that I was in Kansas. It sounded like Kansas. It smelled like Kansas. Very definitely, I was in Kansas.

I had hay fever twice every year – every spring and every fall. I sneezed so badly it was embarrassing. Sometimes I couldn't stop and I would sneeze 10 or 15 times in a row. In class kids would laugh. I figured out how to stop the embarrassment. I just held my breath and the sneeze never came out. It did put pressure on my sinuses and I had a lot of nose bleeds. But, the nose bleeds weren't embarrassing, and nobody laughed when I would lie down on the floor and hold my nose to stop the blood flow.

Dr. Coyle tried a new drug to stop my sneezing. It was called Cortisone. It came in tiny stop-sign shaped light blue pills that I had to pop out of the wrapper. They didn't do much except make me real dizzy, but I still sneezed.

I watched a movie on TV about a man who was taking Cortisone and the more he took the crankier he got. He was losing his temper and shouting at his wife. He finally went to a different doctor who said he was going insane and took him off the medicine. I hoped that didn't happen to me.

"You're catchin' flies, Steve." Mom said that to me often.

"Huh?"

"Close your mouth, Stephen. It's wide open, again."

I thought back to another day when my teacher said my adenoids needed to be checked. I just had my mouth open, and didn't know it. Sometimes it made my jaw sore and it was hard to close my teeth right. I thought I was breathing through my mouth and not my nose that was doing it. When my nose was all stopped up, what was I supposed to do? Truth was – I had spent most of my life with my mouth open, and a lot of the time my jaw was cockeyed, too. My face would get stiff, rigid, sometimes in pain. This was another early MS sign that no one detected.

The summer I turned 13 gave me the opportunity to play in the State Kansas Junior Chamber of Commerce Tournament held in Chanute, about an hour's drive from Coffeyville. It was my first time playing out of town, spending the night away from my family, and being around lots of guys older than I was.

I stayed in a room at the Hotel Tioga with Jerry Wall, but the hotel was full of junior players. After dinner I discovered a lot about how kids spend their time before a golf tournament.

I was in my room cleaning my clubs when Jerry said, "Come on." We wandered the hotel hallways to see what was going on. Some older guys had put beer and ice in their bath tub. Some guys were playing cards. Some were listening to the radio, and playing it very loud.

We saw some guys putting on the hallway carpet on the 3rd floor. They had put ashtrays and glass cups down to use as targets and were playing their own version of miniature golf.

"Hey, guys, come here." It was Mike Scimeca. He was a lot older, but I at least knew him. He was staying on the second floor. He had a grin on his face like he had something devious in mind.

He grabbed a 7-iron out of his bag lying on the floor in his room. He then got a towel out of his bathroom and went to the window. He opened the window and crawled through it.

"Come on, now." His head protruded back through the curtains. "Watch this. F_ _ _in' A. This is going to be so fine."

I crawled outside to see what he had in mind.

"See the bank across the street? I'm going to fly a ball over it. Right over the roof. Watch this."

He laid the towel on top of the short roof which supported the Tioga red neon sign. We were standing on a platform stretching about ten feet out from the wall and twenty feet wide. It surface was black solid tar. It was rough and would have scratched his club. That's what the towel was for.

He put his beer down carefully and put a severely cut Titleist on the towel and made one practice swing very slowly. Eyeing the Chanute First National Bank he swung and hit a ball that flew away and disappeared into the dark night's sky in the direction of the bank.

We listened. No sound. No crashing noise. No broken glass.

"Hah. I did. It. Perfect shot."

I said, "Let me try. I can do that."

"You sure?"

"Yeah. Lemme do it."

He put down another ball, and gave me his club.

It was too easy, Mike said. "Try going over there."

He pointed toward the post office further down the block.

It wasn't as high a roof. The American Flag with the floodlight on it made it an easier target. I took a big breath and let it out. I hit the ball and it flew out there in the right direction into the thin air of night and disappeared.

No sound.

"Whew. I did it. Groovy!"

"Nice shot, Knapp."

The rest of our gallery clapped and we all went inside. No one else was brave enough to try it. As we went back into the bedroom I was glowing inside my body.

I walked back to my room with Jerry.

"I can't believe you did that, Steve."

"I can't either. But, I didn't do too shabby. Did I?"

"Nope."

My score the next two days was decent, but I was far back in the pack from winning. 79-79 was my score. 72-74 was the best score. Andy Neusbaum, a 17 year old, won it. I was only 13. My time would come when I got older. I never hit a golf ball over a city building ever again.

14

7TH GRADE CAME along and I was in boy's choir. We had an assembly where we had to sing for the whole school. We were lined up in the hallway with our robes on waiting for our turn to go on stage. There were other groups in front and behind us, too. My mouth dropped and I gazed at the back of a girl with blonde hair. The hair was especially long and fell down past her waist. I didn't see her face, but no one else could have hair like that in this school.

I kept my eyes open looking for the girl with the long blonde hair. The school wasn't that big. I would find her. I did find her. I had her in a math class, but I sat in the front and she was in the back. I never noticed her before. Her name was Janis Herman. I promised myself I would have to get to know her better. Little did I know that this girl would play a major part in my future. I would have bet $10 against it then. If anyone had told me we'd be married some day, I would have thought they were crazy.

In 7th grade I went to a different school, Roosevelt Junior High School. I took my first class with mostly strangers. I'd been with the same kids for 7 years at Edgewood Elementary and then everything was different. Still, I was pretty sure I would do OK there.

"Get out a piece of paper and put your name on it. I'm going to test you on some of the words we will be covering this semester." Miss Judith Cook, my 7th grade English teacher, had no idea how many words I knew, but she found out that day. She gave us a practice test of 50 words to spell and define. I knew them all.

"100%, uh, uh, Stephen Knapp," she read my graded paper the next day. "Looks like you'll be cruising through this class. Nice going, there."

That year was good and nothing really bad happened to me. I played golf and whatever sport was in season, and just got better and better. By the time I reached ninth grade, I was a starting guard on the school basketball team.

I became more and more aware of my body. I was never going to be a big guy. I would never be able dunk a basketball, most likely. I was starting to combat acne on a regular basis. My smile always bothered me. It was crooked. I smiled regular on the right side of my face, but I couldn't make the left side of face smile the same way. Like it was deformed, or stiff. I could not make the left side of my face smile. It curved down at my upper lip. How could I have ever known it was yet another sign that the left part of my body was affected by MS, and my nervous system was telling me there was something wrong. But, it was not anything to worry about. Everybody had a different smile anyway. Mine just was not symmetrical.

I was a starting right halfback and punter on the school football team. The high school golf coach, Oren Stoner, asked to transfer me to their golf team and I quickly became their number one player, even though I was still in Junior High, and everyone I played against was older than I was. I would subsequently earn four letters in golf, one for each high school grade, 9-12, which put me in a very elite group in the history of the school, since it usually only gave out 3 at the most to any one student. Senior high was only grades 10, 11, and 12. Junior high was 7, 8 and 9. Junior high was in a separate building.

I had a leading role in the school play, "The Double Barreled Detective Story". Janis, the blonde with the very long hair, was in the play, too. We found that we had several classes together every year. We became friends.

I made very good grades. In fact, I was one of the school's best students, especially in math.

Mrs. Colver, my math teacher, pulled me aside one day. She was a gray haired lady, short, but always neat and knew a lot of good stories. She was smart, too. She had a warmth and charm about her that always won people over. She had been in the school system a long time, and was Dad's teach when he went to high school.

"You know I taught your Dad a long time ago, except I was called Miss Clay back in those days."

That really wasn't a question. I knew that was a lead-in to something greater. "Dad had mentioned it to me a couple of times. He really liked you."

"He was very good at math. You would be my best student now except for these silly mistakes. Look at this." She showed me some papers she had graded.

"Eight times four is not twelve. You know that. You added when the sign told you to multiply. Look at this one. One hundred over twenty is not a hundred." She had made big red circles around the ones she was talking about. "Where is your mind, boy? "

She wrinkled her face, cocked her head and looked straight at me. "You always answer the hard questions correctly, but you make these silly mistakes on the easy ones and I just don't get it. Every paper has one or two of these, but there is no pattern. You don't seem to be paying attention every once in a while. You need to be a little more careful. OK? Your scores should be perfect, you know. You're plenty smart enough."

"OK. Thanks. I'll try and be more careful."

I thought I got them all right. I didn't remember making those mistakes. I didn't try to make them. I didn't miss them on purpose. I promised myself to try harder at it. But, that never really happened. I tried to make things as perfect as I could, and I was fast, too. But, for some reason, perfection was not something I could reach out and grab. There were always little stupid mistakes. I guess my natural inclination was to be too fast, and too careless.

My propensity for making "silly little mistakes" would haunt me all of my life, never knowing why I couldn't control them. They would just happen and go unnoticed until it was too late. MS had crept its way into my cognitive processes and I could never nail it down.

Mom liked to stay at home and listen to her albums – "My Fair Lady," "South Pacific," "Gone with the Wind," and the rest of her favorite movie scores. She played the piano sometimes. She'd just pull out the sheet music and play the piano.

She taught me to play solitaire and Canasta and Samba and dominoes when I was younger. There were days when we would entertain each other and listen to music. As I got older we didn't do those things as often. By ninth grade Mom and I rarely spent time together having fun. I think my interests had changed a lot more than hers had. And her time was taken up raising my sister and my brother, Sally and Stuart.

It was typical spring warm and windy day. Our golf team had a tournament in Chanute. We had six players on our team and we got to count the lowest four scores against all the other team's lowest four scores. We would have tryouts to see what order the players would have. Lowest score in the tryouts was "first man" and played with the "first man" from the other competing teams on the day of the match. "Second man" from each team played together and so on. I always played "first man" on our team.

Kansas weather brought wind into the landscape almost daily. In the fall the wind blew the leaves off all the trees and left them bare until spring. In the winter the wind chill could make it feel like it was below zero even though the temperature may only be in the mid-twenties. In the spring the wind proved true the expression"March comes in like a lion and goes out like a lamb."

I liked playing in the wind. It could help me or ruin me, but if I kept my ball low and controlled it, I could make my shots go where I wanted them to go. I'd been playing well in those springtime windy days, but, one day, it worked against me in a way I wasn't expecting.

Besides getting a medal individually I could have won another by being on the winning team. That day at Chanute I had four holes to go and I was in the lead for wining both.

I was standing on the tee aiming at a short par three when, Whack! A ball came out of nowhere, hit the back of my head and bounced past me about ten yards. I immediately put my hands behind my head and bent over. It hurt worse than anything I could imagine.

Where did that come from? My thoughts were answered a few minutes later.

"Are you all right?" One of the players in my group asked if I was OK. It was Warren Wood from Independence.

Boy, That's a real goose egg. Biggest I've ever seen, Knapp."

"I'll be OK. I didn't see it. Where did that come from, anyway? Go ahead and hit. I'm not ready."

I went last. The world had turned suddenly fuzzy. My head hurt and I couldn't see clearly.

"Hey. What the hell are you doing? Why did you throw my ball over there?"

I looked blurry eyed at a kid who walked up close to us while he was accusing me. He wore cut-off jeans and an old T-shirt with blue letters so washed out I couldn't read what it said. He wore a faded blue visor on backwards, and his black socks were hanging around his ankles. He carried his bag backwards with the bottom of it in front of him.

"Do you know how to yell FORE?" - I asked him. Man, I was angry, and in sufficient pain to justify my anger.

"Whaddayamean? What are you talkin' about?"

"Your ball, you nitwit. It hit me in the back of my head. Then it rolled over there all by itself. I didn't touch it."

What an idiot.

"Oh. I'm sorry. I didn't know."

Another kid said the wind was blowing so hard I wouldn't have heard him anyway.

"OK. See ya. Just get out of the way, will ya."

I waited for him to hit his shot and walk off. My head was pounding with pain on the back side and I could feel a huge lump on it. I hit a pretty good eight iron straight at the green. But, I couldn't see the break to the hole very well and three putted for a bogey.

I guess my swing was good enough I didn't need to see very well until I got on the green. I hit good drives and good irons. I putted for birdies on the next three holes, but I went three- putt, three- putt, four- putt. I didn't win the medalist honors. Coach Stoner said I probably had a mild concussion and should have just walked in and told him I was hurt. Heck. I wanted to play and win. I didn't know I couldn't putt with a concussion. I didn't even know I had one. I just wanted to win. I should have won.

Two years later I got hit in the head twice during the summer. Once I was playing golf with Bob, John and Chris Coyle. Chris accidentally hit me with his practice swing and his two iron hit my eye just where the scar is from when GrandDaddy Weiss dropped me on the brass waste basket. The next time I hit myself with a crowbar to the side of the forehead about where Paul Kiser had hit me with his swing in first grade.

I had a summer job loading wheat into a large grain elevator. My Dad was friends with the three owners. Usually I just shoveled it down into a bin from farmer's trucks. But, a few times, I spent the day inside a railroad box car. The door underneath wouldn't slide open so I crawled under the railroad car to pry open the door for wheat to fall. The crowbar slipped. I was a bloody mess walking into the emergency room.

I learned all about butterfly stitches with both of accidents that summer. But, except for a couple of headaches and two scars I was OK. Ever since I had been very young head trauma had been a way of my life with me. On the outside I seemed to have not been hurt too badly. Just some scars to show was all. I never thought once about what damages might have occurred on the inside.

"Steverino," Mom would call me. I think she got that from listening to the entertainer Steve Allen on TV. "You were born with a very hard head."

"Sure was, Mom."

Probably in more ways than one.

"A penny for your thoughts?" she would ask me.

Mom was always asking me that. I guess I looked like I was thinking. I usually was. Maybe having my mouth wide open gave me away. I liked that better than "catching flies," that was her other favorite expression.

"I was thinking about how we learned to play bridge. That was fun. Thanks, I'm so glad you did that."

Mom, Mrs. Martin, Mrs. Beine and Mrs. Wall all played bridge together on Wednesdays. They all had sons about the same age, so for a few weekends the four boys sat at the card table while the ladies stood behind us.

"The main thing is to count the cards. You will not be a good player if you don't count the cards."

"No. Lead trumps. Right now play the king. Good. Now how many hearts are still out?" All of them would volunteer advice whenever they spotted a reason to blurt something out that we might learn about to make us better players.

We learned the rules, how to keep score and how to bid.

It was slow for a while, but they were patient and we learned the game fairly well. Mrs. Beine said, "When you boys get to college you'll be a big hit, all of you will be glad you learned how to play Bridge." Over the years knowing how to play bridge came in handy on numerous occasions. I have always been grateful to the four mothers who taught us how to play, and gave up many Saturday afternoons to do it.

One funny thing was that Mom was left handed. I always copied her growing up. I dealt cards left handed. I could write left handed. I unscrewed tight lid jars left handed. I smoked cigarettes left handed. I vacuumed the floor left handed. I threw a Frisbee left handed. I dried dishes left handed. I even wiped my rear left handed with toilet paper.

15

OVER SEVERAL YEARS growing up and playing golf Dad had made appointments for golf lessons for me with every pro in the area. We seemed to get a new pro every year at Coffeyville Country Club, and I would take lessons from each of them, but we traveled to Independence, Kansas, Bartlesville, Oklahoma, and Tulsa, also, so that I could get better. PGA pros Jack Gibson, Jack Martin, Warren Ryan, Marshall Smith, Jim Pruitt and others, each teacher had some different ideas and suggestions and most of them worked. I practiced and practiced what they told me. I even took a lesson from Jerry Barber who won the PGA, one of the four major golf tournaments each year.

They all said, "Steve, you swing too hard, you swing too fast and you just look stiff over the ball. You have to learn to relax."

One way or another they all said about the same thing. I must have looked pretty unorthodox to them. But, I hit great shots, never the less.

In my mind I was relaxed. There was no way I could be more relaxed. I was feeling a lot more relaxed than what they were seeing, but I couldn't help that. It felt relaxed to me. There wasn't any way to relax more than I already was. It wasn't my fault I looked so stiff.

In the fall our maple tree would drop seeds that covered the ground in our yard. I enjoyed watching them fly as they became detached from the bare limbs and descended, similar to a helicopter propeller going around in circles all the time getting closer to the earth. I called them "whirly birds."

Jerry Wall named my golf swing "whirly bird" because of its follow through. After the ball was long gone and my club was on its upward path towards a nice high over head finish my wrists gave the club an extra loop before stopping. It was something I just developed on my own. A distinctive final maneuver that no one else did. It was my signature follow through on full swing shots. The whirly bird.

Mom signed me up for ball room dancing and Mrs. Ketchum, the dance instructor, said the same thing, I'd been hearing from my golf instructors. "Relax! Relax!" Where have I heard that before? I mused to myself.

"You can't be smooth when you're that stiff." Mrs. Ketchum had a British accent and it sounded like "re-lox" when she said it. Everyone nickered.

My dance partner in her class was Susan Misch. I had known her since kindergarten. Susan never said anything about me being stiff. We did OK together. Not great, but the Foxtrot, the Waltz, and the Jitterbug were not easy to learn, either. But, we both mastered the various steps. Susan had a crush on me once, but I didn't catch the same feeling for her. I never got real smooth at dancing, but I didn't go to many dances anyway.

Besides, how could I have been more relaxed than I already was? I couldn't have been that stiff. How could I play golf and basketball and swim and do everything else so well and be stiff? It didn't make sense to me.

It was early June, a few weeks before my 14th birthday. My golf game kept improving, my scores kept getting lower. I'd been playing and practicing long hours every day. I signed up for a USGA national junior tournament in Wichita, Kansas. If I won that, I would qualify to go to the Nationals.

There must have been over a hundred kids that signed up, and most of them looked a lot older than I was. I didn't know anybody, except the other kids I drove up with. I was paired with a boy age 17 whose name was Gary Bell. He was from Junction City, Kansas.

He was stocky. Wide shoulders. Muscular. His jaw was square and his lips pursed. Crew cut, blonde hair, red sunburned freckled skin. He smiled every so often like he was thinking about something good to himself.

"Hi. My name is Steve Knapp."

"Hi, Gary Bell. Nice to know you. Good luck."

We shook hands. His handshake proved him to have very strong hands. We were in the very last group and had to wait two hours to tee off. I practiced, I putted, and I sat down and fidgeted with my bag and the balls and tees in the pockets. I bounced a ball on my wedge and counted the times before it dropped. Bounce, 1, bounce, 2.....I got up to 98 and quit when I heard my name announced on the loud speaker.

"Now, from Coffeyville, Kansas, on the first tee, Mr. Steve Knapp."

I walked up to the first tee and hit a beauty right down the middle with a little draw. It was going to be a good day. I just knew it.

I birdied the first hole. I birdied the second hole. My confidence grew, but I kept my nerves under control. A few holes later I made a bogey on a par 3, but I eagled the next par five with two good woods and a 30 foot putt.

There was a lot of chatter among groups and we had to wait a lot between holes.

"I'm two under. How are you guys doin'?" I heard one boy say two groups ahead of us.

"I think you're the leader then, haven't heard anything any better," was the reply.

I was two under par also and Gary was one under, but I didn't say anything. Gary gave me a look and made a gesture like he really didn't care what they said. And it might have been just a lot of bunk. We were both playing well and needed to think about just our scores. Nothing else mattered.

On the 17th tee a man in a navy sports coat with a USGA emblem on it asked us how we are playing and asked to see our score card. After studying it carefully he said,"Mr. Bell you are even par, and Mr. Knapp, you are two under par. Is that correct?" We both said yes.

"Mr. Knapp, you are leading the tournament and Mr. Bell you are two strokes behind. All other contenders have completed their play. The best score in the club house is two over par.

Whoa. I knew I needed to bear down and make every shot count. I tightened up a little bit. I hit a bad shot to the seventeenth green, and it came up short. I chipped short and missed my putt. Gary made a par. But, I still had a one shot lead with one hole to play.

The Kansas wind, my ally, was blowing fiercely from my left to my right. I could anticipate the wind would shove the ball to the right so I aimed way left, toward a tree in the left rough, just to have a target, to compensate for the blustery wind. I hit a pretty decent drive. Gary had already hit and his ball was closer to the green than I was. I only had about a hundred yards to the green, but the green was so hard that I was going to have to land my shot in front and let it bounce and roll on. If I carried it on the green it would bounce way over the green. I had to hit a bump and run shot which I had practiced often. I knew I could hit just the right shot.

The greens had been that hard all afternoon. The hot wind had really dried them out and made them very firm. Not nearly as soft as they were in the morning, which I liked much better. In golf I learned to accept what I faced. I had prepared for myself for that shot.

I hit it perfectly. It landed just in the fringe and was right in line with the pin. As I stood there watching and expecting a good bounce up close to the hole, it bounced sideways straight left and it ended up behind a tree to the left of the green. The ground was flat, but there was a sprinkler head in front of the green. It was hidden, but I hit it.

Rats, I whispered to myself. I never said in cuss word in my life. I didn't have any in my vocabulary. But, this would have been a time to use one.

I usually didn't get that mad. I had learned it was better to control my emotions. But, I had no shot at the pin, no shot even at the green. The best I could hope for was to chip close to the green and maybe chip in the next one. I was still in it.

Gary had hit the green and had a fifteen foot putt for a birdie.

My first chip was as close to the green as I could get. My next chip missed the hole barely and stopped three feet past the hole. Bell missed his putt and tapped the next one in. As it stood at that point I had to make my three footer and we would go into sudden death.

As I was lining up my putt, I saw my Dad hiding behind a tree, peering at me. He had his grey suit on and his navy and burgundy striped tie from work. I didn't know he was coming. I didn't expect him to be there. He never told me.

WHAT'S HE DOIN' HERE? I was transfixed on him. Not when I had to make a really important putt. If I made that putt, and if I could win the playoff, I would get to go to North Carolina. If I made that putt at least I would be in a playoff. (I later learned I would have been the youngest junior player in its history to ever qualify for this event.)

I couldn't get Dad out of my mind. I didn't want him there. He never told me he was coming. I didn't want him to see me if I missed. I lined up the putt. I looked at it from three different angles. It broke left a half an inch. It was an easy putt to read.

I stroked it. I pushed it right. I missed it. Two inches to the right. Fast as I could I tapped the next one in.

The man from the USGA quickly approached Gary Bell and shook his hand and announced to crowd he was the winner. Hundreds were there clapping for him. Things were shooting so fast, my mind was spinning.

I thought to myself - I was winning. I was tied. I lost. What had happened? How could it happen? Why was my Dad there to watch me miss that putt? Why did I get such a screwy bounce? Why that time? Why. Why. Why. What could I do now? How could I get that moment back and do it again right? It was hopeless. I blew my big chance.

I was totally crushed. Every muscle, ever fiber in my body was completely drained and exhausted. My brain was empty. My heart was empty.

I had to sign my score card and my mind just went blank. Dazed I shook Gary's hand and signed his card. "Good game, Steve. Tough luck." And I left trying to hide my tears.

When I saw my Dad moments later I yelled at him. "Why are you here? I never want you watching me again!" He had been to most every basketball game and football game and anything else I was ever in, but I was standing there now blaming him. He distracted me. I lost my concentration. I lost the golf tournament. I missed the most important putt of my life.

It was an easy putt. Could had made it five times in a row left handed. After that he stayed away from me when I was playing in any kind of tournament.

Next day, July 10, 1964, Coffeyville Daily Journal headlines on the sports page read "Knapp Barely Misses Trip to USGA Finals." The pain of reading that brought the whole event back into mind all over again.

We moved into our new house two years later than we were supposed to. When Mom got pregnant with my sister they started planning for more room. Our small two bedroom house on Overlook Drive would not be adequate any longer. Mom and Dad spent many evenings talking to two architects – Stitzel & Spitsnoggle. I'll never forget their names.

They designed a very unique home for us, but it took a long, long time to complete. The plan was to have it ready when my sister, Sally, was born. The reality was that we didn't move in until Mom was pregnant with my brother, Stuart, which was almost two years later.

But, it was a really nice house. Made of cedar wood throughout it had a marvelous fresh country smell, and every room had angles that made no room square or rectangle, or like any other room in the house.

During the drawings stage Dad gave me a template and the floor plans one night and told me to make sure all the furniture would fit in the rooms. I carefully laid out all the beds, tables, the dining room table, the grand piano and couches in the rooms where they would go. I must have used the wrong scale because at the time I was sure everything fit perfectly. But, after the house was finished Dad's first comment was about how it came out too small.

"Something is amiss here. The furniture doesn't fit right. It doesn't feel right either." Dad was puzzled. It was tight and not close to the roomy feeling they talked about having.

Not long after Mom came home following Stuart's birth, she had to back into the hospital because she had a hernia from carrying too much weight. With Mom in the hospital, somebody needed to stay with the two babies.

"Steve, this is Wilma." Dad had brought her over to our house. Wilma was thin, pretty, dishwater blonde, about 35, and carried a suitcase in with her. "She'll be staying here a few days until your mother is strong enough to join us again."

"Sure. OK. Hi, Wilma. Nice to meet you."

A live-in nanny. We never had one of those before. I had no idea where Dad found her, and how he got her so fast.

The next day I had a chance to talk with her. I was on my way out for school, and she was in a bathrobe and drinking coffee smoking a cigarette in the kitchen. I exchanged small talk with her for a few minutes and then I asked what was really on my mind.

"Wilma. How do you know my Dad?"

"Oh." She paused and took a puff on her a cigarette. "We met at the Southern Club. I work there, you know. I wait on tables at the bar. This is just a part-time thing for me to help y'all out."

She stayed for four days. Then Mom came home, weak, but at home. What I didn't figure out until later was how perfect that situation was for Dad. She was more than just a bar maid. Dad had become a regular customer at the Southern Club after work, after lawyer stuff and after his radio performance nights. It took a while for me to put it all together. Now I knew why he was always coming home late every night, and why he was drunk sometimes. Even though I was skeptical we never talked about it. I should have, but I never asked him anything really personal.

"Are you OK Dad?" I came home at 12:30 am on a Thursday and he was sitting in the dark on the sofa smoking a Camel when I walked through the family room on my way to bed.

"Yeah, I'm OK. Go to bed, son."

"Night."

I found him there often, always in the dark, late at night. There was a layer of smoke that hung about three feet off the ground. His ash tray was full. You could a glowing ash on the tip of his cigarette. His glass was full of scotch. Must have been things weighing heavy on his mind, but I didn't know what they were.

I was elected President of the Student Council. Janis gave a traditional rah, rah speech about school values. Stuart Read gave a pretty good speech that made a few kids laugh. Mine was especially clever and masterful and I was extremely proud of it. I practiced it over and over in my head all night the day before. I mentioned different teachers and talked about hypothetical impossible situations like building a monstrous huge structure in shop class that no one would want to steal. The speech worked. Dad helped me write it.

A few days later Dad and I rode to school together. Roosevelt Junior High School was old and was made of red brick, probably material made long ago right here in Coffeyville years earlier when it had five large brick plants that were fed from natural gas wells. When the wells were exhausted the plants closed. Many of Coffeyville's streets and sidewalks were laid with home grown bricks.

We had eaten lunch at home. We listened to Paul Harvey on the radio and he was about ready to drop me off when we heard the announcement that President John F. Kennedy had been shot in Dallas, Texas. He died soon afterwards. That day, marked forever in America's history, was November 22, 1963.

The Principal of our junior high school, Mr. Kenneth McClure, was a friend of Dad's, and a fellow former Naval officer who drove with him to reserve meetings a few times. He called me at home that night and asked me to prepare for a certain poem he would ask me to read to the student body the next day. After a short speech he gave, which I didn't hear because I was so focused on what I would do next I read a very solemn rendition of "O Captain! My Captain!" by Walt Whitman, and we were all dismissed for the day.

I was 14, and Dad got me a great job. He was friends with the manager of KGGF, the town's only radio station. They were losing all their young announcers to the draft for the war in Viet Nam. I was too young to be drafted, and we were never going to move out of town, so I made a good choice.

I had a mature speaking voice. (It changed in seventh grade. I was the only bass in boy's choir that year.) The radio station just had to train me. I was one of the youngest radio announcers in the country, but I didn't know it then.

Early on I announced a story about a man who won an award after he died, and it was awarded posthumously. I learned the hard way about mispronouncing words.

"It's pronounced pahst-chu-mus-ly, not post-hume-ous-ly." Ed, my trainer for the night, was very precise and demanding. Nothing I did got past him. He was a little rough on me, but I did learn from him.

"Sorry, I didn't know that one."

"Then look it up before you go on the air. Don't make that kind of stupid mistake again!"

My training wasn't always smooth, but I got the hang of it eventually. They taught me how to read and talk, speak distinctly, and put the right emphasis on the right syllable. I broke sentences up into phrases or groups of words that sounded well together. They taught me how to breathe at the right times, and how to pause when it was appropriate. They taught me how to sound professional. I used my voice with its wide range of inflections to help convey the meaning of the message and the material I was reading. I garnered many lessons and skills there that served me well long after I left the radio business.

"Remember this, Steve," another older announcer named Steve Osinga told me one day, "A lot of listeners out there don't know you are reading this stuff. But, they believe what you say because you are saying it on the radio, which is sacred. So you have to sound like you know what you are saying is true. They are counting on you for the truth. Don't ever let them down."

I took Osinga's words very seriously. Always.

There wasn't any one person who taught me. I sat with whoever was on duty and learned how he did things. I was the object of collective wisdom. Everyone had a few good things to add to my repertoire. I took a few points from six or seven different men and added that to my own style to make a pretty decent announcer after a few months.

I played records, commercials, non commercial spot announcements, I learned how to keep a log, or make the right connections to patch into a live Kansas City A's baseball game. They taught me to play pre-recorded programs with a big Ampax reel-to-reel tape player about religion, or crop statistics, or how to live a better life. We were a small radio station, but we were the only radio station in Coffeyville, broadcasting to the Magic Circle. That was an audience of about a half a million people living in southeast Kansas and northeast Oklahoma.

"You are listening to AM Channel 690, Coffeyville, Kansas, on your radio dial." I had to say that every 30 minutes at the top and bottom of every hour, and write it on the log. Most of the job wasn't hard. I just had to do the right thing at the right time. Preparation and timing were keys to everything.

I talked to all the different kinds of people who listened to me. Farmers, and ranchers mostly, but a lot of other kinds of folks, as well. All different ages. Working men, retired men, housewives, professional women, kids, you name it. Probably a lot of horses and cows and pigs and dogs and chickens listened to me, too.

I played records by the Beatles, Dave Clark Five, the Everly Brothers, Frank Sinatra, Elvis Presley, Roy Orbison, The Kingston Trio, Dean Martin, Perry Como, the Mamas and the Papas, just to name a few. A real mixture of tunes, for sure. But, we had to appeal to everyone's interest, so I had to play quite a variety.

The best part of my radio job was that I had to put together a fifteen minute newscast and I had to start it exactly at ten o'clock. I pulled stories from two wire service machines, Associated Press and Reuters, that spit out paper like crazy, but they were the source of all the state, national and international news. Then, I got weather forecast information, current readings and any new stories from the fire department. It was too much usually, and I had to shorten it, organize it, and make it sure it all flowed together to sound smooth and professional.

I was always on top of all the current events. At eleven o'clock I played songs for a program called Moods til Midnight, and then after the National Anthem completed exactly at midnight, I closed the station and went home. I closed the station three or four nights a week. The job lasted for four years until just before I graduated. I really liked it. It helped me develop many skills and gave me self confidence that aided me greatly down the road. My ability to express myself to others, my talents in public speaking and having the confidence to organize materials and present them has paid dividends over and over throughout my career.

When I first started, I worked along side another man until they thought I was ready to be on my own. One of my favorites to work with was Rodney Lay. He also played in a band, and later went to play in Roy Clark's (Laugh In) band, but he was always nice and fun to be with.

When I started smoking, Rodney let me because he smoked, too. I was amazed at how he could blow smoke rings and that was one of the reasons I started smoking. I thought that was cool. Especially, when he blew one smoke ring and then blew a second one that shot right through the center of first one. I thought how cool was that? I had to learn how to do that, so I did. I just needed to practice.

The control room at KGGF was perfect. There were windows on three sides, but it was a very small room, just big enough for two people to sit in. There were two turn tables to play the records, two tape players for the commercials, and the big Ampax reel to reel tape player on the back side. It was 100% quiet in there and there was no air circulation, so smoke rings could slowly float out of my mouth and widen out ever so slowly as it drifted across the room before it finally lost its shape.

Dad had started working at the radio station also, but in a different way. He and Bob Pratt announced football and basketball games for the Coffeyville Junior College teams.

Dad did the "color" for the games. Before the games he would interview coaches on both teams, he calculated the statistics and gave them at half time and at the end of the game.

"Well, hello there, thanks Bob. This is Charlie Knapp. In the first half the Red Ravens shot 38% as a team on making 14 baskets out of 36 attempts and adding another 6 points from the charity stripe......."

He quickly earned the nickname "Slide-rule Charlie."

He carried a small white slide rule in his white, cotton, button down shirt pocket with him next to his Camels and used it deftly for all his statistical calculations.

The second job working radio took him out of the house and on the road half of the games. He and Bob Pratt, who did the play-by-play, traveled all over their conference area which took in south eastern Kansas and northeastern Oklahoma. He did it more for the fun and excitement than the money, which he said wasn't much. Or, maybe it was an excuse to get him out of the house late in the evenings. If they paid him like they paid me I believe him. I made federal minimum wage, $1.25 per hour.

Dad bought Mom a new shiny 1965 Ford Mustang convertible, light blue with a white top. I had to wait six months after I got my driver's license before they let me drive it. Then it was my car to use sometimes when Mom let me use it. I thought it was cool to smoke and flip ashes into the air when the top was down. The world was my ash tray then.

Dad was invited to drive it in the Annual Christmas parade, and a few months later he was asked to drive it in the high school home coming game at half-time. He loved to show it off even though it was Mom's car.

Of course, I wanted to show it off every time I had the chance. I gave Janis a ride in it and we just drove around the town. I'm sure she was impressed. The coolest thing to do was drive through the A&W root beer stand. You didn't stop. You just drove through it and then back out onto 8th Street going the opposite way. I could cruise up and down like that for hours. One night I put about 200 miles on that car and never once got out of the city limits, which was only a few miles in any direction. That didn't go over so well when Dad noticed it.

I skipped school one day and gave three girls from school a ride to Wichita and back. It was a two hour drive each way. Janie Misch just had to see a boy friend and I just wanted to do her a favor. Unfortunately, lots of unforeseeable things went wrong, indicating severe lack of judgment, but doing a nice favor seemed to be all that was important at the time.

All three of their mothers checked out some rather fishy stories about spending the afternoon with their sick friend and called the school. By the time we got to the Wichita city limits a Kansas highway patrol car pulled us over. We were all identified and all the parents were contacted and comforted, but punishments would be issued separately after we arrived back home.

We saw the boy friend, Jack Marnell, for a brief time and headed back. It was not my lucky day. About 5 miles outside of Coffeyville, I had car trouble and had to pull to the side of the road. I started waving to the cars as they passed by. David Sisler, a senior in high school, gave us a ride into town in his pick up truck, and took us all home. Coffeyville was like that, lots of friendly helpful people. In small towns everyone knows everybody. Sometimes that's a good thing.

Dad called a tow truck. I was grounded for a month, except for going to work and school. He cooled off, though. A little.

"Stephen, you know better than that. Why did you do something like that?" Mom and Dad lectured me with right and wrong every so often. I knew right from wrong when I was about 4 years old. Sometimes I did the wrong thing anyway. I knew I could get by with it, or I wanted to see if I could do it and not get caught. It was always a conscious decision. A measured, weighted choice. The penalty if I got caught on one side and the thrill of doing it on the other. I never meant to hurt or injure anyone intentionally. It was kind of a personal dare. I approached many situations similarly. Once in a while I got caught somewhere along the way. But, not always. Mom had convinced me nothing bad would ever happen to me, so why not take a few chances?

I might have been a cognitively affected poor decision-maker, or just an undisciplined youth who had to learn from his own mistakes, rather than exercise good judgment. I became an anomaly to a lot of people. "Surely he knows better. What's the matter with him?" I could hear their thoughts and read their faces even if the words were not spoken close enough that I could hear them. But, I didn't care.

I walked outside and sat on a lawn chair in the back yard. I wondered why I always got in trouble just trying to do something nice for someone. I didn't mean to get anybody upset.

I sat and watched the sun dip beyond the horizon and disappear into the wheat fields across the street. I could hear a symphony of sounds, coordinated like an orchestra, but only the percussion was playing, no melodic music. All I heard were the locusts, the crickets, the grasshoppers and the birds. The warm, moist atmosphere sprinkled with dust and pollen from the Elm trees and the wheat fields added a familiar backdrop. The lightening bugs made no sound, but they certainly added illumination to the production. It was a unique kind of natural harmony, and I could sit and listen and absorb it for hours.

I could especially smell the wheat from nearby fields further down the street. I could smell the freshly cut Bermuda grass of our back yard's morning trimmings. This was Kansas. I loved Kansas. Why couldn't I fit in and do the right thing in Kansas? What was wrong with me? Was there somewhere else I could be different?

Dad came out and snapped my thinking back into his terms. "Son. Take a look see. What do you think of this?" Dad showed me a picture of a putter in a magazine." Golf Digest," our favorite monthly magazine.

"Looks interesting. I think I'll order it," and he did.

Dad was always in search of the "perfect club" to improve his game and lower his handicap. He and Dr. Coyle spent hours experimenting with the latest "new theory" on golf found in Golf Digest magazine. He was never satisfied with his game. Neither was I with mine, but new theories didn't excite me. I believed in harder practice. The thick calluses on my hands were a testament to my longs hours on the driving range.

When the putter arrived, I thought it looked weird. There was an inch of opaque plastic between the shaft and a very odd looking putter head that had deep flange behind the putter face.

But, after a few strokes, I decided the sweet spot felt good. Dad said to give it a try it, so I did just that.

I took it with me to my next tournament in Garden City and it worked great. I one-putted the first ten holes. I wasn't playing well, but making putts every hole made up for a lot of bad shots. I was one under par to that point.

Then I had this thought. *What was I doing? No one made every putt. Sooner or later I was bound to miss one.* One the next hole I four-putted the green and my score for the rest of the day was rendered to a mediocre 75. At least I could dip the new putter into the hole and with a little jerk make the ball fly up into my hand without having to bend over. That was a neat trick in and of itself. I liked little tricks like that.

16

I'M NOT SURE what happened first or how it started. I sort of lost my popularity with my friends, and I spent a lot of time with new friends, older guys. I played pool a lot at the pool hall. I started drinking beer. I was smoking cigarettes, Marlboros. My grades weren't as good. But, I didn't care. I was going to college and I was going to have a successful life. Doing what I didn't know, where I didn't know, but I was sure it was going to be OK. My life was always OK.

Mom told me over and over, "Get that degree, Steve." I knew I would. I never thought much about what I would study, or what I would do for a living. I knew it would work itself out when the time came. I never questioned the fact that I would always be able to do the right thing when I needed to.

Mom and Dad were not getting along most of the time. I had a baby sister, Sally, and a baby brother, Stuart. I wasn't home very much. Mom had a house keeper, Christine, to help her with the kids and the house. Working at KGGF, playing golf, school, pool hall, going out at night. I was a busy guy.

In the last year I played football on the school team coach, former KU star Jim Jarrett, talked me into playing. I was afraid I might get hurt and ruin my golf chances. I was a junior with two more years of high school. I was hoping for a golf scholarship as a possibility in college. He convinced me I was going to be OK, and he said I was the best punter in the school. I agreed. I also caught passes on some plays, some plays I played defense, but mostly I was a kicker.

My legs were short, spindly and I couldn't jump forward out of my shadow, but I could run all day long, and I could kick a foot ball into the next county. Well. Not that far, but farther than anyone else in Coffeyville. Never could understand the disparity. I had some weird legs, for sure.

It was a crisp cool autumn night. There a twinge of frost on the ground and I could see my breath every time I exhaled. I could even form smoke-ring-like shapes with my breath, but they didn't hang in the air nearly as long as the real ones. The ground sparkled as it reflected the night lights overhead. The stars were out and a sliver of the moon, like a smile tipped sideways, stood high in the eastern sky. It was a perfect night for a football game.

We were playing Parsons, another small Kansas town in the Southeast Kansas division, at our stadium. Parsons had a tight end that was a foot taller than I was and probably outweighed me at least 60 pounds. It was in the third quarter, we were behind 12-zip, and I was in the defensive backfield guarding against the long pass. I played on both sides of the ball, offense and defense. I lined up right across from him and he had this cocky look in his eyes. Obviously, he looked at me like a wolf eying fresh meat.

I could see the quarterbacks focus on his target and the ball was spiraling in my direction. I jumped high and hit him just as he caught the ball. We collided, joined together, revolving in the air, and he landed on top of me.

Ooooof. I got him. That was all I could remember. Then I passed out.

They put me on a stretcher and carried me to a spot behind the bleachers and made me sniff something so awful it made me come to. There was a crowd of kids around me waiting to see if I was alive, I guess. As I started to move they cheered. I felt really good about that. They cared.

"I'm OK," I shouted. I waived my hand to no one in particular. My eyes were still blurry. Chalk up another hard hit to my head.

I got up shaking, and somebody helped me slowly make my way to the locker room. Things were foggy but I changed clothes and found my Dad waiting outside the door.

"Are you OK, son?" He seemed very concerned.

"Yeah. I'm fine. Let's go home."

I probably had a mild concussion that night, but I was OK. I guess Dad never thought about taking me to a doctor. There must not have been a doctor at the game. If there was he did not come to me. I shuffled into the house and collapsed into bed. The next morning I was fine except the foul smelling salts lingered in my nostrils.

Yuck.

The next week I set a school record with a 65 yard punt. But, I didn't play any more defense. I caught a few passes and made a few runs as a half-back in some of the next games, but mostly just kicked, which was fine with me.

The fear of not being able to play golf started to dwell in my mind, especially whenever participation in other sports came up. I knew golf was my best sport, and each year guys got bigger, faster, and taller compared to me. At 5' 8" and 140 pounds, I was a shrimp swimming with sharks and it was just a matter of time before I was going to have something really bad happen to me if I continued to press my luck. Playing football or basketball on a school team no longer captured my desire. It was too risky.

Winter came and we had our first snow flurries just before Christmas. Dad had accepted another offer to drive the Mustang in the town's annual holiday parade, but it wasn't to be that year.

I was driving home after closing the radio station. The snow had semi-melted and then iced over again creating a slick glass-like road surface. I had never driven on anything like this. I knew to go slowly, but I didn't know the breaks would lock up. I hit the Fourth Street Bridge going no more than 15 miles per hour, and smashed the front end of the shiny blue Ford Mustang. Nobody told about driving on ice. Another lesson learned the hard way. It was another strike against me in my dissolving trust from my parents.

Golf was my equalizer. Men twice my size and strength could not hit a golf ball as far as I could, most of them anyway. Plus, I could score better and hit all kinds of shots. My puny size didn't matter. It was what I did with it that counted. I expected I would be among the best players all of my life. I had that much confidence and I loved the game. I was certain I'd be playing all my life. The great thing about golf is anyone can play it at any age.

I went on to tie the course record, a 6 under par 66, at my home course at Coffeyville Country Club. One Monday, the course was never busy on Monday because the clubhouse was closed, I played 72 holes that day and walked the whole way, carrying my bag on my shoulder. I was only 15. I won many golf tournaments all over the state of Kansas and Oklahoma and did pretty well in the ones I didn't win. I had accumulated over 25 large trophies and tons of medals which are all nicely displayed in my bedroom on my shelves. I had earned a reputation as one of the best players in Kansas. I was very proud of that and took a lot of confidence from it.

Janis and I never seemed to be on the same page at the same time. In the 9th grade I thought she may have had the hots for me, but I wasn't interested in her as a girl friend. I was going with Doris Kinsch. Sophomore year we reversed rolls. I had fallen head over heels in a love with Janis, but she was going with Dallas McKellips. She was nice to me, but not too interested in the same way I was. I had a crush on her at that point, but I could only hang on so long before I looked elsewhere.

I sprained my ankle badly in gym class and couldn't wear a shoe for three weeks because it was so swollen. I danced with Janis once at a concert at the top of Memorial Hall. Even though she was going with Dallas, she gave me one dance. It was painful but worth it.

Memorial Auditorium opened in Coffeyville on Armistice Day, 1924. It was a beautiful three story structure of brick and limestone with six Doric columns facing the east side. Coffeyville Junior College played their basketball games there and sometimes special functions would use the building for their activities. Dad did a lot of radio announcing there.

Once when I was a Boy Scout I was in the Memorial Hall building with hundreds of other scouts for a big convention. I played the part of a pretend TV cameraman and I pushed around a large camera looking device on wheels that Dad had made.

With Janis that night I could only dance slow dances because any pressure on my ankle really hurt and I couldn't move very fast. Slow dances with Janis was fine with me.

Junior year we had a few fun times together, but nothing serious. In Coffeyville everyone had a reputation. Mine had fallen on bad times. I smoked. I drank beer.

I got caught in a few lies trying to make myself sound better than I was.

I shot snooker at the pool hall. My friends from a few years ago acted cold to me now with good reason. I was a social outcast. A pariah.

My reputation was so bad it was hard to find nice girls to date. Janis distanced herself from me for her own social protection, I think, but she was still friendly to me.

Senior year we were too busy to get a handle on our feelings for each other, but the spark was always there.

I was feeling sad, alone, rejected, and not doing anything that I could brag about outside of my golf accomplishments. I fit nicely into the shadows. I didn't see people and they didn't see me.

I was walking into the gymnasium, taking a shortcut on my way to a class, and there were new decorations just put up for the pep rally that afternoon. Purple and gold crepe paper streamers, twisted around and around, were hanging anywhere they could find a place to attach them all over the gym.

I felt angry and hurt. I pulled down several of the streamers and ripped them apart. I never told anyone I did it. I walked out and no one saw me. I knew it was wrong, but I felt no remorse about the mess I left behind.

On my way home from school I saw a girl getting out of a car and she shouted to the driver and started walking.

"Hey. Want a ride?" Who could resist being offered a ride in a 1965 Mustang convertible?

"Who are you, yeah, well, I guess so." She was cute. Young, but nice looking. Never seen her before in school.

"I'm Steve. Please to meet you. I don't want to pry, but you weren't too happy getting out of that car just now. You looked like you were mad enough to rip somebody's head off. Right?"

"Yeah, well, you know…. That's used to be my boy friend, but not no more. I've had it with him. I'm through with boy friends. They're all so stuck up."

"I'm not stuck up. Not all guys are bad, you know. You maybe just got a bad one. It's like fishing. Sometimes you have to throw them back in the water. They're not one you want to keep. They're not for you."

"You think so? Man, you don't know him. He's rotten."

"Then you are better off. Maybe it just took you a while to see what he was really like."

"You're right about that. Where do you live? What grade are you in? I'm Beverly" We sat and talked in the car on the side of the street for an hour and I took her home.

Soon Beverly and I were seeing each other regularly. Although she was four years younger than I was I enjoyed being with her, except when I wanted to do something else.

"Bev. I can't go out tonight. Not tonight. I'm going to be sick. Not sick like you get sick. I get really sick.

Any time the moon is full I change for the worse. Beverly, I get crazy just before a full moon."

"Oh, really?" She was so very worried. "Why?"

"I dunno. I just live with it. I mean, man cannot live with bread alone, but I deal with it."

"OK. I get it bread. Hah."

She didn't get it. I was playing with her mind. I was kind and generous and polite with her, but not always honest. I don't know why. I played on her sympathy.

I didn't take advantage of her, either. We just kissed and made out. We laughed a lot. I needed that. I escaped to another world when we were together. It was just the two of us. A made up fantasy world, but it was comfortable.

We adopted a song by Johnny Rivers called "The Poor Side of Town." That was our song and we turned up the volume and sang it together whenever it played on the radio.

Bev and I went up to Big Hill often. It was the highest point of elevation in the area, and it offered many nice private places to park a car and sit with a girl friend.

"Tell her no, no, no, no....." the Zombies were singing on the radio. I didn't have my KGGF on, they had a Kansas City A's baseball game on. I had WLS, Chicago, turned on. I liked it better when the reception was clear. They had all the latest and best music.

As we took the curves to get to the higher, and quieter, more private areas, my mind started to wander. The music was getting further away and I was drifting into in a trance. It was like I was drowning, but not in panic. I was trying to get to the surface, slowly. Like swimming, but not getting any closer. I kept reaching. I was kicking with my feet to the beat of the music.

"Steve, watch out!" Bam. Bam. Bam.

Beverly tried to warn me, but I was asleep at the wheel. I awoke but too late to react. I went off the road, down a ridge, and after hitting two low branches the car smashed into a tree trunk and came to a very sudden halt.

"Bev. Are you OK?"

"Yeah. You scared me. I'm really, really scared."

"I'm sorry. I fell asleep, I think. Oh, God. Oh, God.

I'm in trouble now. What am I going to tell Dad? I can't talk my way out of this one."

We listened to the radio and held each other. I didn't think to realize Chicago was in a different time zone, so when I heard the famous DJ, Dick Biondi, say 8 o'clock I thought it was 8 o'clock where I was, but it was really 9 o'clock in Kansas, and I was about to be an hour late to work and didn't know it.

The car started up, but it sounded like a thrashing machine. It limped back to town to the radio station parking lot. I hoped nobody noticed the awful racket, but I'm sure lots of people did. I was in big trouble again.

Hal, the radio announcer on duty sat in the control room there with his wife, rolling his knuckles on the counter clearly quite angry at me for having to wait an extra hour for me to show up. They were madder at me than Dad was when I got home. I woke up Mom and Dad driving in. I probably woke up half the neighborhood, too.

Hal and Mrs. Hal took Beverly home for me. They weren't mad at her, just me. I was the trouble maker. I was the one who was late.

The next day I flunked a trigonometry test I hadn't studied for. Things seem to be going wrong in bunches. Life was not going too swell at that moment.

GrandDaddy Weiss wrote me a letter telling me how I needed to be more careful driving. His mechanical engineering degree must have come in handy for him. He quoted the equation for centrifugal force, Mv^2/r, and it followed with an explanation of how it applied to my car and circular momentum. I'm sure Mom asked him to write me.

I never did remember to thank him for that old watch.

I wasn't going too fast around a curve. I fell asleep. Pure and simple. No one believed me. At least we weren't hurt and in two weeks the car got fixed like brand new again. That car had been hit almost as much as my head, but not quite.

17

ONE OF MY best friends that I played many holes of golf with was Jerry Wall. His Dad played with my Dad on Thursdays and Sundays. We caddied together growing up. We played golf together for many years. We had a good rivalry all the time. We'd be on the practice putting green and I'd say, "OK, this putt, this 15 footer, is for the Masters. I'm Arnold Palmer. I make this and I win."

"I'll bet a bottle of pop you don't make it."

"You're on."

I stroked it. Missed.

"I'll make it this time." Clunk. It went in.

"Two out of three, Jerry?"

"Nah. I'll go you all the way around the green, 18 holes, and I'll play you. I'll play you for a bottle of pop and the Masters Championship, to boot."

"OK. Flip you to see who goes first. Heads or tails?"

We spent hours on the practice green, putting, chipping, competing against each other. Sometimes when it was too dark to see because it was so late, we were still out there putting, waiting for our parents to pick us up. We just kept practicing.

A bottle of pop only cost a dime, Dr. Pepper, Fanta Grape, Fanta Orange, Coke. It was all just a thin dime. Jerry bought me a lot of pop every year. I usually was a little bit better putter. At least a scosh. Sometimes more than a scosh.

He would have fits when I won too often. He would carry on and on, and I would razz him, but it was all good fun.

"What's a matter, Jerry. Forget how to sink a putt?"

"Shut up. I'll get you next time."

Next time seemed to always repeat itself, but he did beat me often enough to keep him interested.

Jerry became my partner in high school golf. Our combined score was usually better than most other teams and we won many medals together. I was usually a few strokes lower than him but several times we finished 1-2.

The hot days of Kansas summers never bothered me. It could be over a hundred degrees and I would feel great. I never wore a hat. Hats bothered me. They distracted me. And, if they're too tight, they hurt. Years later, when I had to wear a hat at in the Air Force, my head would hurt and I would get a headache and I'd get a line all around my head where it squeezed my skin. If I wore it loose, it fell cock-eyed or dropped on the ground. There wasn't any in between way to do it. Besides, I always looked stupid wearing a hat. I think my head was just the wrong size for hats.

That's wasn't just me talking either. Jerry Wall once said, "Knapp, you look stupid in a hat." Exact words. I'll never forget them. Didn't matter if it was a golf cap, a visor, a wide brim hat, a baseball cap, or even a stocking cap, I just looked stupid wearing it. Needless to say, I rarely ever wore anything on my head.

I think the hotter it got the better I played. I was stronger and looser, and even though I sweat a lot, I could handle the heat.

I went to the golf course every day during the summer. When I asked Mom – "Can you take me to the club?" Typically I heard, "Not right now, honey. I have an errand to run. It'll just a few minutes. Want to go along?" She always smiled afterwards and raised her head like she really wanted me to go along and was interested in my response.

"No. That's OK. I'll walk."

I had learned not to trust Mom on this point. One errand meant one, and then another and then another. A trip to the post office to buy stamps would, after talking to Jean Berryman, Winona Beine, and a few other friends standing in line, would take her to the Karbes grocery store for some carrots and lima beans. Then on to Newberries for a bridge club gift for Ada B., and back to Jack's Texaco service station for some gas and a car vacuum.

It may not stop there. She might run all day. She never did one errand. And a few minutes was never in her real timeframe. A few minutes stretched easily, too easily for her. I don't know if she ever realized it. Several hours was more like it. I didn't want to follow her all over town, and I didn't want to get upset. I mainly wanted to be at the golf course and to not be with her.

Too many times I had gone along with the "oh, just one quick stop" thing. She always made me late when I said yes. I hated that. I couldn't stand to be late. And, I really couldn't stand it when somebody else made me late because they didn't share my same value of being punctual. Being late with Mom was a given. It was no big deal for her.

It was for me. It was worth the three mile walk to the club not to ride shotgun with Mom all day.

"Sorry. I'll pass."

Life in Coffeyville was a constant slow pace, no rush. The older I got the more I realized how the whole town seemed to be in slow motion. No one was in a hurry, ever, and it drove me nuts.

The walk to Coffeyville Country Club started in Edgewood which was the housing division on the west side of town; however, to get there most of it was walking along a hilly two-lane country road. Eighteen wheelers drove by every so often and stirred up the dust like a huge force of wind that came out of a blast furnace. I didn't mind. It was far better walking there than going shopping with Mom.

Oh, I just have one stop to make, Stevo…. That drove me crazy. No thanks. Those words made me shiver.

It's not like I was expected to be there at any certain time. Jerry and I had no set time, and the course was seldom busy enough to need tee times. But, wasting the day with her was just that – a wasted day. I couldn't practice and play and get better if I wasn't out there doing it.

I had a crooked smile, a stiff body, a head that seemed to get hit a lot, but I was OK. I had a lot going for me. Even though the town was slow, the people walked and talked and thought slow and I was stuck there until I left for college it wasn't bad. Life was actually good. People would tell me, "If you have your health, you have just about everything that is important." I had that. I was in super good health. There was nothing wrong with me.

18

I WAS OUTSIDE so much I became very observant of weather patterns and changes. There was a spot on the horizon in the northwest sky. When dark clouds started rising up just at that point, it would bring rain in a few hours. If the dark clouds were south or north of that point the rain storm would go around us. Funny how it worked that way, but it always did. I could tell with amazing accuracy if and when it would rain.

Most storms moved quickly and in an hour or two it would clear up and be nice again. They say, "If you don't like the weather in Kansas just wait a short while and it will change." That saying held true most of the time.

I liked to watch the lightning that would come along with the storms. In Kansas the sky is vast. No tall buildings. No sky scrapers. No towering trees. No mountains. I could see for miles and miles in all directions.

When lightning streaked across the sky it was amazing how far it would split like the branches of a tree and just keep stretching farther out as it kept on splitting into smaller fingers. I saw lightning millions of times, but I never had a bolt get close to me. Maybe I was just lucky. I wasn't scared of it. I understood lightning. I could predict it, too.

Dad told me how to count for lightning. When I saw the flash I began to count – one thousand one, one thousand two, one thousand three, and on, and on until I heard the thunder. It's roughly a thousand feet for each second I count, so if I get to a thousand ten, then the lightning was about 2 miles from me. That's because sound travels slower than light, and the thunder travels at about 1000 feet per second. 5000 feet is about one mile. 10,000 feet is two miles. My gauge is two miles. If I only got to nine seconds or less I would seek safe shelter. The lightning was too close, and it could be very dangerous. I spent hundreds of hours outside. I became a close friend of Mother Nature. I think I knew Her pretty well.

Once on the 9th hole I sliced my drive deep into the right rough next to a crabapple tree. As I approached my ball which was sitting up in the high thick Bermuda grass, a bird attacked me. It flew at me, circled around and flew at me again, shrieking. It was a red-winged blackbird, with a beautiful red triangle underneath its wing. It flew at my head several times before I realized it had a nest with baby birds chirping and she did not want me around. I left my ball there and walked back to the fairway and dropped one down. That was her space and she didn't understand I was just playing golf. I wasn't a threat to her, but there was no way to tell her that. So, I kept my distance.

Another time I walked along the lake water's edge on the 9th hole looking for balls. The algae growth was heavy and the only way to find balls was to stir up the water with a wedge and lift up the green plant life to see if any balls were hiding there. It was a natural landing spot for many an errant shot, and not too many players would make the effort to dig through the water and muck to find their ball.

Something moved underneath my foot! Yikes! I jumped up and stepped back onto the bank just in time to see a small snake slither into deeper waters. Herb Wilson warned me Avie Shlacher, who played every single day, said that Cotton Mouth snakes had been seen in the lakes. I got to see one up close, but I didn't get bit. I guess we were both scared of each other and we quickly went our own ways, and fortunately for me, in opposite directions.

I was playing the same hole another time and was standing quietly on the tee box, right next to an old dead tree that got hit by lightning a few years ago. I had missed a putt on number eight and I was angry. I tapped my driver against the tree a few times. A dozen yellow and black bumble bees flew out of the tree and came after me!

BZZZZZZZZZZZZZZZZZZZZZZZZZZ.

They chased me until I walked backwards down the bank and fell into the water before they went back into their tree. I'm sure they were thinking, "serves you right, Bucko." At least I didn't get stung. Mother Nature taught me many interesting lessons on the golf course.

Jerry Wall and I played many rounds of golf together. We swam together, ate together. We were like brothers at the club. Always together. We talked about most everything and anything that came to mind.

One day Jerry said, "Hey, Steve, let me ask you something."

"OK. What's that?"

"I've always wanted to ask you this. Why do you shake your hand like this?" He motioned his left hand like it was loose and waving, or maybe like the wind was blowing a sheet hung on the clothes line.

"I have no idea," I told him. "I don't think I do that. When do I do that?"

"All the time" he told me, frowning incredulously. "Several times daily. When you're playing. You mean you don't know? I can't believe that. It's all the time."

"Your kidding. I truly have no idea what you are talking about. I want you to tell me the next time I do it. Prove it. OK?"

I couldn't imagine I was doing something that odd and not know it. But, he was around me so much he probably knew my actions better than I did. It's hard to see yourself, especially on the golf course. I believed him, sort of.

It didn't take long before he caught me. "There. You just did it. You waved your left hand." He told me a few more times that day when we were playing, but my hand had already moved back down to my waist so I couldn't tell if I was doing it or not. It must have looked weird when I did it. Not only did I have my mouth open most of the time, but, I waived my hand, as well.

Who would ever think I had MS? I had never hear of it before back then. I doubt anyone could have connected my aberrant behaviors with MS in 1964 anyway, but I'll never know.

Jerry and I drifted into the pool hall down town. The air was smoky. There was an acrid, dusty odor that made it hard to breathe. "You've Lost That Lovin' Feelin'" by the Righteous Brothers played on the juke box.

"F..... you. Damn it. Pay me."

"Draw it straight backwards. Only way to make that one and get shape."

"Frozen on the rail, Babycakes. How do you like that leave, Man?"

"Rack 'em."

I learned a lot of new vocabulary along with learning 9-ball, 8-ball, and Snooker. Most of it I never used, though. I became hooked on the atmosphere. It was competitive; it required skills I needed to work on to get better. Pool was a lot like putting, it took good aim and a soft touch. The guys were friendly, and it didn't cost much to play.

The owner's name was Frisbee. He always spoke to me. He was friendly. It became a new hobby for me. For me it was a great place to escape. Heck with the tarnish it brought on my social standing.

Life was good in almost every way, except for Dad drinking a lot. He drank Cutty Sark straight, sometimes a whole bottle in one night. I knew. I emptied the trash.

And glass items had to be separated from the rest of the trash. Home life was becoming a place to avoid, and I did so as much as I could. I babysat my little sister and brother when Mom and Dad went out. Otherwise, it was see ya later.

Dad signed me up for the Annual International Orange Bowl Junior Golf Tournament in Coral Gables, Florida. The golf course was located next to the famous Biltmore Hotel. I practiced every weekend, no matter how cold it was. Even if it was 35 degrees outside and windy, I was at the club hitting balls, putting, chipping, getting my game ready for the two day tournament right after Christmas. Of course, our club had no sand traps or Bermuda greens, so I wasn't completely prepared when I got there, but I was as ready as I could be. I was very motivated and wanted to do my best.

Florida was beautiful and the first day I played great. I shot a 72 and was tied for second place in a field of over 300 kids from all over the world. I was happy with that day, and reporters and photographers spent time with me after the round. I told them how I practiced with 20 degree wind chill conditions and frozen ground. No. We don't even have sand traps at my course, but they did have a putting green. I answered their questions for over thirty minutes. I'd never gotten so much attention, but I liked it. I saw the article in the Miami Herald sports section written about me the next morning. I got a lot of print.

The next day I was paired in the last group with three fine junior players. The first was Johnny LaPonzina, touted Golden Boy of junior golf. His picture had been on the cover of Sports Illustrated. The second player was Bobby Cole, former Master's Champion Gary Player's protégé, and he won the British Amateur three months later. The third player's name I forgot, but his home course was the Augusta National, in Georgia where the Masters is played. And rounding out the group was me, Stephen Knapp, Coffeyville, Kansas. Boy, did I feel outclassed.

I remember comedienne George Goble said one time on TV,"It's like everyone else is wearing tuxedos and I am an old brown shoe." I was in a very elite group and it was a big adjustment. It was a totally new experience for me.

Although I drove the ball past them all on nearly every hole off the tee, I clutched and couldn't hit a green or make a putt. They were older, bigger, taller, and more experienced. There was a gallery of about 500 people following us, which was about 499 more than I was used to. I shot 82 and had to settle for 20th place. It was a good experience, and it was my first trip to Florida.

I never would have expected to live there later on in my life. Never in a million years would I ever think that was possible. Florida was like being in another country, a million miles away from Kansas. Odds were I'd never be close to there again.

I went on to win many golf tournaments in high school and was the State JC champion when I was 16. I won by 8 strokes over the next best score. I played in the national event in Houston, Texas. I played with Andy North and Lanny Wadkins, both of whom advanced later on to be very successful PGA pros, and TV golf commentators. I didn't play well in Houston. My score was decent, but not great.

My golf game was as good as I could get it at 16. I could hit the ball high, low, straight, hook with a curve to the left, slice to the right. I had a great short game. I once had 7 putts for 9 holes, including two chip-ins. I hit the driver extremely long for my small frame and short height. The wind became my ally and I used it to my advantage. I was always happy when the wind blew, harder the better, because I knew I could play just as well as when the air was calm, which gave me a competitive advantage.

I had spent hundreds of hours practicing on the dry, ground-cracked, dusty, not manicured, sparse grass driving range at Coffeyville Country Club. It wasn't fancy. I used my own practice balls and had to pick them up with my own shag bag. When I was the only one there practicing, I could see the pattern made after all the balls were lying on the ground close to my target. They dotted the sunburned brown Bermuda grass like buckshot in a scatter pattern. All of them were pretty close together. It didn't matter much if I hit a 9-iron or a 5-iron, the pattern was about the same.

I had long ago toughened my hands to the point I had calluses on top of calluses where my hands applied pressure to the club's grip. I had long since endured the hands bleeding and the pain of blisters. I still used Gauzetex to tape fingers when a callus would tear away and expose raw flesh. I accepted pain as a necessary evil of dedication to my practicing. I was never going to let pain keep me from putting in the practice time I needed. I didn't wear a glove. I wore them out too fast and didn't like them anyway. I didn't wear a cap either. Hats and gloves were not my cup of tea. I also didn't wear socks, not playing golf. They got dirty quickly in the Kansas dust bowl and I liked the lower tan line. I hated it when cockleburs would stick to my socks and it pricked my fingers to remove them. There was big difference in color between my white feet and my deeply tanned legs.

I practiced in all conditions – windy, hot, rainy, cold, frozen ground, and nearly dark. I played in all these situations and was not deterred by any of them. I practiced with my ball on flat dirt, divots, tall grass, next to trees and shrubs. I could hit a 3-wood 250 yards off a flat dirt lie and make it go anywhere I wanted it to go. I could do it all. Or, at least, I thought so.

I never paid for practice balls. I had plenty of them, hundreds, in fact. Most of them I found by wading through the four lakes on the golf course. Steve Adudell, a friend of Dad's, gave me all his Maxfli golf balls that he had put big cuts in. He only played with new ones and when he bladed a shot and made a gash in the ball, he replaced it with a new ball. I had a lot of brand new balls with creases in them, but they made good practice balls.

When I wasn't on the golf course, I was thinking about being there. In school my hands would be together like I was holding a club. If I was standing, I would unconsciously start shifting my weight from the right to the left foot. In the restrooms I would stand in front of the mirror and watch my form as I pretended to make a swing. I focused on the position of my hands at the top of the swing, if I had kept my head still, or if I swung back slightly inside or straight back. I lived and breathed golf even in my sleep.

Dad said Jack Coyle and he were going to sign up to play in the Kansas Men's Amateur. It was in Topeka that year. He asked if I felt like going with them.

"Sure!"

We got the forms filled out and sent them in. Dad paid for both of us.

We finished playing our practice round at the Arrowhead Country Club in Topeka, Kansas, and went back to the Holiday Inn to clean up. Dr. Coyle turned on the TV.

"This just in…...A tornado has been spotted in the southwest part of Topeka. Indian legend has it that the hills there are sacred tribal burial lands and the spirits will protect all who live in that area. But, just in case, please be advised to seek shelter if you are in that vicinity."

"Hey. I think we are in the southwest part of the city! Dr. Coyle had a better sense of direction than I did. No surprise there.

Dad contemplated his next thought. "Let's look outside."

He opened the door and there it was coming toward us. A black and gray swirling monster. It was two thousand feet across at the base extending straight up on both sides. No wimpy funnel. It was huge. I thought at first there were sea gulls flying around it, but I what was looking at was the debris it had picked up.

Dr. Coyle ran to the car and got his 8 millimeter camera and started filming it. (He later sold the footage to the National Weather Service.) I stood gazing in awe of its size. It wasn't anywhere close to the funnel shape I expected a tornado to have. I'd only seen pictures of tornadoes and heard stories. This was the "real McCoy."

"Let's get inside, Steve. We may need to crawl under the beds." Dad was obviously nervous, and cautious. It was probably the first time since he'd left the Navy that he'd been in any kind of threatening situation.

The tornado veered away from us and in a few minutes in was gone. As far as we were concerned, we were safe. The sacred hills got hit hard.

All of Topeka was in turmoil. The powerful deadly tornado headed for the downtown area and dissected the city, mowing a path of destruction for miles. The damage was of historic proportion.

The tournament was postponed the next day. The city was in shock. Streets were impassable. Downed trees, parts of buildings and houses were leveled, debris and destruction were widespread. Dad and Dr. Coyle elected to return to Coffeyville. I stayed on thinking I had a good chance to win. I bid goodbye to them and spent the day with friends I'd met from other tournaments. We walked around looking at the incredible damage.

"You see that over there?" We were talking to a man sitting on a side walk. I didn't respond. I just let him talk. He was dressed in jeans and a T-shirt, barefoot, unshaven and clearly depressed.

"That used to be my business. I was a printer. It's wrecked so bad I'll be lucky to, no never mind. It's totally unsalvageable. It's a total waste."

"You see that building over there?" he continued and he pointed across the street. It was impossible not to listen to him. It was a three story apartment building, windowless, structural cracks running down the front side and I could see right through it to another damaged building behind it. There was a bed hooked by one leg hanging out over a window sill.

"That's where I used to live. I'm sure it will be condemned when they get around to look at it."

"Wow. That's terrible what are you going to do now?" I asked him.

"One more thing," as if that wasn't enough bad news. "You see that pile of bricks over there?'

Just down the street parts of a brick building seemed to have come apart and restacked themselves in piles. "My car is under that pile, that one right there."

Crunched blue metal stuck out on one side of the heap of brown bricks and mortar. The two story building next to his had completely apart and it had made several piles of wreckage in a big mess.

"I have no job, no business, no place to sleep and no transportation. My whole world just got blown to smithereens. I'm goin' to catch a bus to California. Start all over. Nothin' here for me. Nothin'."

"Good luck, Mister," we offered, but there was little solace.

There wasn't much else to say to him. I felt sorry for him. We walked on.

We saw a seven story building that looked like a typewriter turned up-side down. Each story was shifted a few feet closer to the street. We saw stacks of cars picked up and discarded back to earth like broken toys. Ten or more on top of each other.

We saw a small airport where more than a hundred single engine private planes were partially or completely destroyed. The news spoke of at least seventeen people reported dead and more were missing.

One of the most amazing sights, which I had heard about before, but was skeptical until I actually saw it, was the pieces of straw, and twigs, and grass that were sticking sideways at right angles into telephone poles. The awesome power of the tornado left a large album of destructive pictures which will be inculcated into my memory forever.

The tournament did start the next day and I was ready to be on the fairways and off the streets which were still reverberating from the devastation.

I birdied the first three holes and then the wheels fell off, and my day turned into a disaster of its own. Instead of qualifying into the championship flight, perhaps being medalist on the first day, I finished with a horrible score of 84 which put me in First Flight.

The following rounds were match play and the next three days I breezed easily through winning by large margins. My game came back and I was then in the wrong group, really. It looked like I sand-bagged the first day, but I didn't. It was just a sorry, rotten way to start for me.

Sunday, I had advanced to the championship round match. The winner would be the first flight Kansas State Champion.

I met my competition on the first tee. "Hello. My name is George Carver. This my son, Ben, his wife, Loretta, and my three grandchildren. I hope if you don't mind them tagging along."

"Pleased to meet you. All of you." They nodded politely.

George was the one person I had to play against to win. But, it turned out differently than I expected.

George was about 65 years old. Seasoned with a dark tan that spoke volumes of years of being outside in the hot summers and strong Kansas southerly breezes, playing golf daily, probably retired, probably a very good player. He had white hair, a large frame and a continuous perpetual smile which I never got used to looking at. Worse than that - he had a family that was totally faithful to him.

We flipped a coin. He won and hit a perfect drive straight down the fairway, about 220 yards. His family clapped and collective voices shouted "Good one, GrandDad."

"Way to go."

I out drove him 60 yards. No one clapped for me. There was only silence. George grabbed his pull cart and the family army followed behind him a few steps. I walked alone.

George hit a 3-wood onto the front part of the green. I hit a 9-iron just inside of his ball. We both two-putted. This sort of play set the tone for the day. He didn't hit it very far, and he didn't make many birdies, but he was straight, accurate and his short game was outstanding. He could have gotten it up and in from the ball washer, except he was never that far off line.

He was unbelievably steady and consistent. He smiled to his family all the time. We never spoke. I wasn't just playing him. It was me against the family – George and his gallery. I was by myself against the crowd all alone. He had played thousands of rounds and knew the course backwards and forwards. I was playing him on his home course. I was the stranger, the underdog, the unknown, a high school young whipper-snapper. They didn't know me from Who Laid the Chunk. I was just another guy that GrandDad would knock down, carve up and whittle away until I collapsed. I was the enemy.

They didn't know who they were up against.

I made par on the first hole, then birdied the second, then three putted the third for a bogey. I was long, occasionally crooked, and not very consistent. I blew some easy shots. Our games were total opposites. He won a few, I won a few. However, after 18 holes we were tied. I swear I beat him in every way, but we were tied. So, we went to the first hole again to play sudden death. First one to win a hole won the whole thing. That's how it worked.

He hit his usual 220 yard drive straight as a string. He probably came close to being in the divot from his drive that morning. He was that automatic.

I hit it directly over his ball 50 yards further down the fairway. It rolled another twenty yards after it landed. I was in an ideal place to get it close to the pin.

It had become annoying to hear the encouraging words from his gallery which always followed every one of George's shots, no matter if he hit a good one or not. I was hurt that no one was there to root for me. It was deadly silent for my shots regardless of whether I hit a great shot or a terrible one. It didn't matter at all.

He knocked his second shot with a 5 wood on the green 15 feet from the pin. My second shot, a wedge, nearly struck the flag, but I hit it a tad hard and it disappeared into the trap behind the green. First trap I had been in all day. I had seen George get out of two of them and both times he put it about a foot from the hole. I could do that I thought as I walked to my ball.

I had to. I couldn't let him beat me. Of course, I'm sure he thought exactly the same thing. I was thinking to myself. "I'll get it close and par. He'll miss his birdie putt and we'll move on to the next hole. It's a par five I can have a good chance to beat him there."

Then I came back to reality. "Oh, great." The lie in the sand was terrible. My ball was up close to the lip of the trap and it was not going to be an easy shot. There wasn't much room to work with between me and the hole. But, the lip wasn't too high. I decided to putt it and take my chances.

George was eyeing his putt, not paying me much attention. On the face of it the advantage was his. Nine times out ten either he would make it, or I would fail to get down in two. Either way, he would win. He still had that insincere smile on his face that by now had me going so much I couldn't stand to look at him. I putted.

Bam!

It hit the flag stick squarely and dropped into the bottom of the cup. Maybe it was lucky. Maybe I hit a great shot. It didn't matter. It went in. I made a birdie.

The silence had never been more deafening. I had to control my excitement. There was no one to share it with. In one quick stroke the balance of pressure had shifted.

No one there could appreciate the difficulty of the shot I had just made. I got my ball and stood to the side watching. The pressure had turned 180 degrees. For the first time it was on George now.

"Come on. Sink it. You can do it. This is your time."

His family gallery did their best to wish it into the hole for a tie, but it was not to be.

He left it short. He quickly walked up and tapped it in, picked up his ball and the flag stick and jammed it in the hole, turned and headed for his bag.

"Let's go. That's it for today." He slammed his putter into his bag and began walking.

That's all he said. No congratulations, no nice round, no nice shot, no hand shake, no nothing. We all walked back to the club house in agonizing silence. No one said a word. I had to restrain myself. I couldn't express the feelings of victory I'd desperately earned. I was a gentleman. I was a good sport. I almost felt guilty that I had won. I had defeated the man, the family, and his pride.

They were indignant without saying a word. The body language of the adversarial group sunk to its lowest depths.

It was the most unpleasant win of my life. I had never been more emotionally drained. I left Topeka with a large trophy, and a lot of stories to tell about a deadly tornado and my unusual shining moment of suppressed exuberance.

19

WARREN WOOD BECAME a true friend whom I met from playing golf competitively. He lived in Independence, Kansas, 18 miles to the north of Coffeyville, and we played against each other many times in school matches and summer tournaments. I beat him more than he beat me, but not by much. He invited me to spend the summer with him at his home and Mom and said OK.

He was taking two summer school courses at his high school, so it made sense that I should, too. I took typing and driver's education. It was weird going to classes where I didn't know anyone. Actually, I did know a few of the guys because I had played against them in basketball or football. But, I'd never really talked to them or met them on any social level. All the girls in my classes were complete strangers. After always knowing everyone for their whole life, this was a unique experience, and a good one.

I didn't make any close friends because I left with Warren at the bell and we headed for the golf course. He would turn the radio on in his car and usually" I Can't Get No Satisfaction" by the Rolling Stones, or "Turn, Turn, Turn" by the Byrds would be playing. It seemed every day it was one or the other.

Warren and I walked toward the first tee. We'd finished school for the day and figured we could get in 18 before dark.

"Hey, remember when you and Jerry Wall, David Gaughn and me played last month?"

"Oh, Yeah. Jerry and I lost because you called out "driving contest!" on the seventeenth hole and I took the bait. I blistered one right out of bounds. I nearly hit a horse grazing in the pasture. That two stroke penalty made the difference between us winning and losing. Is that what you were talking about?"

"Hah, Yeah. When we on the seventeenth again, I'll give you another chance."

Warren was taller and stronger than I was, and he was a year older. But, when I caught one solidly I could drive it past him. Jerry Wall was my high school two-man partner and David was his partner. We played several matches against each other. It was always a good time, a great lasting rivalry.

We played our way around the Independence Country Club course in a good rate at arrived at number 17. "You're on. It's driving contest all over again. Go ahead. You go first. Show me what I need to beat."

"OK." Warren hit a beauty. It went on his usual trajectory. It started low, faded slightly to the right and traveled far and in the fairway.

I hit a low hook and it started like it would go out of bounds again, but swerved back to the left, easily in the fairway, it and bounced several times well beyond his ball.

"OK. You win that one. Nice drive. But, it didn't match the pressure of the last time"

I hit my shots with a slight draw. My natural shot starts a bit right of the target and moves from right to left. The wind was blowing right to left so it favored my shot. I beat him because I drew the ball, and he hits his with a slice swing curving it in the opposite direction.

It was the wind that made the difference.

"Yeah, well. We'll have to save that pressure for another time. I guess, so. But, at least I didn't kill any horses. That's pressure, you know."

We both laughed.

We became good friends playing golf. There was always the underlying competition against one another, but there was respect and camaraderie, as well. We could stand there on the range and hit balls and eat dust and be perfectly happy together. Our sense of humor seemed to mesh well.

"So, how's the typing going?" He was taking some advanced classes so we didn't ever see each other in school.

"I've pretty well established my speed/accuracy threshold."

"Huh? What in the heck is that? Pray tell?"

"It goes like this – If I type 30 words per minute I get a nearly perfect, zero error, grade. But, I if I kick it into high gear and type, say about 40 words per minutes, then I make about ten mistakes. Faster I go, the worse I type. Hard as I try to change it, that's how it goes. Speedy fingers will never be my forte."

"You know what?" He adjusted his very worn, salt lined navy blue visor.

I leaned closer to him.

"What?"

"Well, when you speed up your backswing, like you did trying to win our driving contest, you know the one with Jerry and David? " I knew exactly what he meant. "You don't do as well. So, driving and typing are the same for you. Better wise up and keep it under control."

"Thanks. Thanks a bunch, Warren. Now you tell me!"

We both laughed again.

In many ways that was a great summer we spent together. I didn't get into a trouble. I didn't make anybody mad. I learned to type and drive a car, so I could get my license. And I spent some time getting to know a guy who was like a brother to me. He was an only child, and I was, too, for the first 13 years of my life, so I guess it was a time we both needed to share with each other.

My stay with Warren and his Mom and Dad ended after the Annual Independence Amateur Golf Tournament. It was the biggest tournament in south east Kansas every summer. It drew players from Kansas, Oklahoma, and Missouri.

Warren and I signed up for the Championship Flight. We were going to play against the best field, the top amateurs, the best competition around the area.

I saw Jim Bullard from Ark City on the putting green. I knew he was good just by his reputation. This was going to be a fun day. We would all play 27 holes and the lowest score won. Simple as that.

I was paired with two men I'd never met before. One was from Wichita and I never heard where the other one was from. But, they seemed nice.

"Now on the tee…Mr. Steve Knapp."

I hit last and then we were off.

It was a nice day to play. Hot, windy, humid. Perfect for me. I played well. After 27 holes I was even par, and I was tied for second with three other players. Bullard was the winner and was 3 strokes better than anyone else. So, a four man playoff was next.

Second in a regional tourney with a pretty decent field was not too shabby for a 16 year old kid. I think I raised a few eye brows when I teed off for the playoff. My age and my small frame stood out from the other players.

We had a gallery of several hundred. It was neat. I could hear them talking.....He's so young? Where is he from? He must be good. I've never seen him before. "

I just kept walking toward my ball. My pride blossomed. This was cool stuff and I loved every minute of it.

One man bogeyed the first hole and there were three of us left.

We all parred one, two and three. Not in the same fashion, but that didn't matter. Just the score, that's all that counted. It's not how pretty, it's how many.

I began thinking, "If I made a 3 on the next hole and they all made 4's or higher, I'd win second place." That's the best I could do, I decided to go for it.

I didn't even know what the prize was for second place. I couldn't care less, I just wanted to win.

The fourth hole was a par four with a blind shot off the tee. I couldn't see the green, but I knew exactly where it was. The hole was not that long. I could drive it in one and take two putts and win. That was my plan.

I had played this hole about 30 times and I'd never come close to the green, but that day I thought might be the day if I hit the right shot.

I swung too fast. I swung too hard. I'd already played 30 holes and I was probably a little tired. And there was pressure, although I scoffed at that notion. Pressure from the gallery. Pressure from the players and the competition. Not really. I thrived on it.

In golf there are a few things you never want to do. One of them is to duck hook a drive into trees to the far left of the fairway, and have the ball roll down an embankment where after you find it sitting on top of a tree root you discover you have no shot toward the green. Good players would try to avoid that, but not me. Not that day.

I double bogeyed the easiest hole we'd played so far. I lost. A guy name Otie birdied the hole. He won second. The other player parred. He won third. I was fourth.

Much to my chagrin, fourth place won nothing. Nada. Zilch. Not one iota.

I walked off, bag on my shoulder, ready to call it a day. I was exhausted. And dirty. Crawling down that side hill to get to ball got me all covered in dust and I had a thousand little stickers called cockle burs clinging to my socks. I had worn socks just to look nice for the tournament.

I picked the wrong day to look nice and wear socks.

"Hey, there, M-i-s-t-er S-t-e-v-e K-n-a-p-p. He said it real slowly. Over here if you will, please." A man, I had no idea who he was, waved his hand at me.

"Hi. Uh, Yes, Sir. What's up?"

An older gentleman, probably in his 60's, white beard, very tan, dressed nicely in plaid shorts and a soft yellow Chemise Lacoste shirt with a little green alligator on his chest spoke to me in whispers.

He cut me off and edged my way far enough from the crowd that was still lingering around the putting green. No one could hear us as we walked. He wanted it that way.

"Let me tell you straight away you played a superb round of golf today. Magnificent, and at your age, you've got quite a future.

Stay with it, young man." He had a recognizably Scottish accent. I knew that much. "That wedge shot you hit on 9th hole, the way you played the terrain was brilliant. Set up a great birdie for you. Very impressive."

"Thank you. Forgive me, sir. What's this about?"

"I'm John Macintosh. Pleased to meet you." He held out his hand and we shook.

"If you were a wee bit older you could have been walking off the grounds here with having won a new Wilson golf bag. Full sized you know. Jim Bullard won the new set of Wilson Staff irons. Second and third place each won a MacGregor set of woods. You should have gotten the new bag. Fine bag it is. But the Committee didn't want to jeopardize your amateur status with your high school or whatnot. You could get in a lot of trouble down the road and we didn't want that. For your protection, you know, son? Do you understand?"

I nodded. I never thought of it, but I knew he was right.

"Still, I think you should have won something." He held out a sleeve of Titleists. Three new golf balls.

"I know it's not much, but this is for you. Off the record, you see. From me. Don't tell anyone now. Go ahead take it."

"Thanks. That's very nice of you."

We shook hands again and exchanged goodbyes.

I felt funny. I played good, great in spots, but I made a stupid decision on the last hole. My chances of driving that green were one in a million. Three balls – that is more than I deserved. But, it was nice of him.

I'd been gone six weeks. Home, Coffeyville, life in the family, however, hadn't changed, and when I returned, it was as if I'd never left.

In the latter stages of my senior year everything was starting to fall in place. My focus has changed and it was all about dealing with the future. Golf would have to wait on the back burner for a while. My Dad had helped me get, through his association with Kansas Congressman Joe Skubitz, an appointment to the United States Air Force Academy in Colorado Springs, Colorado.

My math SAT scores fell a little short of Air Force Academy standards. Those stupid little mistakes were still affecting my life, so I went to their Prep School. But, it was still a college education, no tuition, five years in Colorado and then flight school after that. One day I would be a commercial pilot. Sounded pretty good to me. My future looked very bright. I would be "The All American Boy." It was my destiny.

I thought back to the American Airlines trip I took solo when I was only ten and the captain showed me all the dials in the cockpit. I could do that. Sure. Why not?

Dad would never say things in simple straight forward terms. But, he always had an obscure way of getting the point across. Mom said he had a dry sense of humor.

He told me a joke once about a prison where all the inmates had known each other so long they had all heard each other's stories a million times. So, they assigned numbers to their favorite jokes, and skipped the time having to tell them over and over.

A new prisoner had just come in and they told him about their system of jokes. His cellmate said, "Just call out a number. See what happens. Forty Eight!" All the men guffawed and roared for several minutes.

"Go ahead. Give it a try," he offered.

So, the newcomer yelled out "Ten." But, there was silence.

"Try another one, son."

"OK. Twenty Three!" Again, only silence.

"Sorry, kid. I guess some can tell 'em and some can't."

John Wall and Dad had just finished playing the eighteenth hole and went to the 19th hole for a game of pitch, which was the usual routine for them.

"Hey, Charlie, I can't find Jerry. You seen him?"

Jerry had put on quite a bit of weight over the last few years, and had we called him "whale man". No one could possibly not see him if he was in the area of your sight.

"No. I'm not sure. I'm not sure if I saw him or not. I did see a total eclipse of the sun standing on the high diving board at the pool just now. I guess that might have been him."

That was the kind of classic standard remark that only Dad would make.

I had to go take a physical exam and do a rigorous set of exercises including timed running short distances, throwing a medicine ball and several other activities. It was part of the qualification standards I had to meet to be accepted into the Academy. I had to travel to Oklahoma City to an air force base there and stay for two days.

I returned midday and went back to attend my last class. Spanish with Mrs. Lydia Butterfield. She was a very exacting teacher, and let me have it when I sat down.

"Steve Knapp. You are a disgrace. You smell like a smoke stack. Your feet stink, and you just don't seem to care about anything. I know you are about ready to graduate but, you better get your life straightened out, young man. You need to make your parents proud of you."

I usually slept in her class, and that day, and following a two and a half hour drive, I'm sure the scent of smoking a half a pack of Malboros in the car all during the trip lingered in my clothes. I didn't wear socks all the time, but when I did, my feet itched, and I scratched my feet in class. I took my shoes off and rubbed my feet. I could tell the kids around me cringed and whispered when I did that.

After I arrived at home from the radio station on a Wednesday night I heard this awful grinding noise outside and I went to see what it was. It was Dad driving his car, a beige colored Chevy Impala convertible, and the front end was severely crushed in.

"I have to go back," he told me, and he got his coat out of the hall closet and started walking down the street. It was about 30 degrees outside and it was about 12:30 at night. I grabbed my letter jacket and walked out the door to follow him. I had no idea what was going on, but I had to find out.

"Wait, Dad. What happened?" I ran after him.

"I think, I'm pretty sure, I think I hit something. I have to go, I have to go back." His speech was slurred and he didn't act normal.

We walked together in silence for three blocks. I could see flashing lights ahead of us. He stopped close to the curb at the Alter's house, and his breath heavily rolled out of his mouth in the cold air.

"Mr. Knapp, Charlie, is that you? I need to see you over here." A policeman wanted to talk to him alone, and I kept my distance. Obviously, they knew each other. I guess that helped, but I wasn't sure what would happen next.

Dr. and Mrs. Alter were standing outside in their pajamas wearing winter coats over them. He was a veterinarian. He did the work on Dana's ears years ago when she was a puppy. A light pole was knocked over, and some shrubs were mangled in their yard. I quickly figured it out.

I talked to the Alters and they confirmed my thoughts. They didn't know for sure who did it until Dad and I came back. They had already called the police who was preparing some paperwork when we arrived.

"You go home, son. I've got to go with him." He nodded toward the policeman.

"Right. See ya later."

That was just great. Dad was drunk, hit a bridge and ran his car into a neighbor's yard as he caromed off the bridge. Then he drove off and went home. I guess he felt guilty and went back before he got in trouble. Maybe it took him that long to realize what he had done and sober up enough to think it through.

I was so hurt and embarrassed I didn't know what to do. I didn't want to go home. I didn't want to go to school. I wanted to disappear. If I could have just melted into the street, I would have right then and there. I didn't know what I wanted, but it definitely wasn't this.

I felt stupid standing there as the Alters looked at me.

Dad's car hit the 4th Street bridge, lost control to the left, jumped over the curb, hit the light pole and was finally stopped by the bushes. Somehow he backed out and screeched his way home, disturbing many folk's sleep along the way, I'm sure. It was too noisy not to.

At a little after 1 AM, I walked downtown to the Coyle's house. I'd watched my Dad drive off in the back seat of the cop car. I was mortified.

I knocked on their front door. All their four Weimaraner dogs, kept outside in their fenced in back yard, barked like crazy.

"Hi, sorry to wake you. I know this sounds weird. Can I spend the night with you?" I was noticeably in tears. I couldn't hold them back.

I gave them a quick summary of the night's events. They graciously found a bed for me in a guest room and I spent the night there. Mrs. Coyle called Mom to let her know where I was, and that I was OK She may have not heard about Dad, either. I spent the next three nights there. I was so embarrassed and ashamed I felt like I had no home any more. I couldn't accept what had happened. But, Mom talked me into coming back. She promised it would be different.

It wasn't just Dad's wreck that bothered me. The relationship between Mom and Dad had become unbearable for me.

I was being used as "the sneak". I was a spy for both sides. It was too hard to play both roles and favor both sides equally. Mom would tell me to check on Dad. "Go find out if he's over there at Wilma's house. Just see if his car is in her driveway."

Dad would say, "Don't tell your mother where you found me. I'll talk to her myself. Let me handle her."

I couldn't take it anymore.

One night Dad came late, took his suit jacket off and all kinds of mail fell out of his pocket. I stood silently watching while he grabbed the envelopes and stuffed them back into his pocket. He looked at me with a guilty expression, like I'd caught him doing something wrong.

"There are three months of bills here, Steve. I don't know where I'm going to get the money to pay for them. I carry with them with me until I figure out a way." Then he went and poured a drink for himself and lit up a Camel cigarette.

Many nights I came home from the radio station and Dad would be sitting in his chair, smoking in the dark. I could see the lit ember move around in the air as he flipped ashes into the ash tray. He was wearing his pajamas and just sitting quietly by himself. Smoke hung like a cloud across the room indicating he'd been there a good while.

I couldn't see in the dark, but I could guess there were a dozen or more cigarette butts in the ash tray.

"Dad. You OK?"

"Sure, son. Go ahead to bed. I'll be there soon. You need to get some rest."

"OK. G'night."

I just wanted out. Or, for my life to get a whole lot better fast. I didn't know how to handle it. My sister and brother were affected, maybe more than I knew, but I thought I was getting the worst deal. I figured it dug deeper into me. They were still young and didn't know what was going on. I knew Dad was fooling around on mom, right here in town. I wondered if she had done the same to him in Michigan.

I usually go to sleep quickly, and stay asleep all night without waking. I guess I stayed up so late my body needed rest when I finally give it a chance to have some.

I dreamt, but nothing unusual until one morning when I awoke to the scariest dream of my life. I've probably had 9,999 dreams that left me in my sleep or passed out of my thoughts soon after waking. But, one dream I had during that time in my life has stayed with me to this day in my conscious memory as vividly as the night I had it.

Somehow I had found my way to San Francisco and I was on the Golden Gate Bridge. I had made my decision to jump and end my life. I planned it, thusly. I would exhale as I was falling and empty my lungs of air. As I hit the water I would take in all the water I could into my lungs and let myself sink to the bottom of the bay.

I jumped off and started descending. Slowly time passed as I fell, I was getting closer to the water. I saw many people in my life pass before my eyes. They were all frowning, or acting disappointed in me. Then I hit the water.

In that split second of time, as I found myself plunging deep into the water, I changed my mind. I wanted to live. I knew that no matter what life offered me in the future, it had to be better than what it was then, and I had to stay alive to see how it turned out. If it was, indeed, going to get better, I'd better stick around to enjoy it.

I climbed to the surface, stroke after stroke, holding my breath. Determined to live. Determined to see another day. A better day.

As I reached out, stretching my arms to their maximum, to break the water's surface. I could feel their choppy waves and I could actually inhale air again, I awoke from the dream. I had made it, and I lived, but I was scared. Awake, I was terrified as to what I had just dreamed. God, it was real. I thought it was happening to me.

Just as if captured in an old movie, I have replayed that dream over and over in my mind hundreds of times. I can still see the bubbles in the water.

I didn't need an analyst to figure out what that was all about. I was glad I lived in my dream. I was relieved I had changed my mind. I was encouraged that things might just get better if I just gave it a chance. When, or where, I didn't know. But, somewhere out there was a better life for me. I had to endure my present circumstances until it changed. It wouldn't be long. I could do that.

My brother, Stuart, was only 4. He'd been crying a lot. He would stand and grab Mom by her knees and beg for her to pick him up. It was like he could feel the unhappiness in the air and wanted more comfort and security. I knew how he must have felt. Worse than me. At least I was getting out soon. It would be a lot longer for him.

Dr. and Mrs. Coyle had a great family and they were always nice to me. They were always happy and laughing. I played a lot of golf with three of their sons – Bob, John and Chris. The Coyles were like a second family to me. Sometimes they invited me to go with them out of town, to Bartlesville or Tulsa. We always joked and had a super time.

I went with them to see the British hit band Dave Clark Five perform that weekend in Tulsa. That was a time I needed them worse than ever. They were like the older brothers and family I never had.

Things simmered down at home after Dad's accident. Uncle Frank, who was also an attorney, had to bail Dad out of jail. My Dad's an attorney. My Dad was supposed to do that for other people. Dad was supposed to be the good guy who helped the bad guy. The whole thing didn't make sense and I just wanted to get as far from it as I could.

The best thing about going to the Air Force Academy was it was a long way from home.

I started to prepare myself for my new adventure, but it wasn't quite time yet. I still had a few more weeks to go to graduate.

One Thursday night at KGGF a bunch of kids stopped by about 10:30. I was in the room where they had a grand piano and I was playing to my own enjoyment my version of "Stand By Me" by BB King.

I had just started an album of soft music for the Moods 'til Midnight segment of the evening programming, and I had a few minutes to myself before I had to go on the air again. I was all alone. All the other employees had gone home hours before then. I looked out the window and saw a bunch of kids by the glass front door waiving their arms trying to get my attention.

"Hey, let us in. Amy needs help. Come on Knapp. Come out here."

I walked into the lobby and stared at them from behind the locked door.

"What's all this? What are you guys.....? I can't let you in"

I didn't let them in. I was the only one there, and security rules prevented it. I knew all of them, and they were not really friends. I just knew them at school. But, they had a girl with them, Amy. I knew her, she was a friend and she was too drunk to stand up. They propped Amy up, sitting and leaning on the glass front door and left.

I felt trapped, and sorry for her. I couldn't leave her where everybody in the world could drive by and see her leaning cross-legged against the front door. What if she stood up and fell down the steps? I waited until they drove away and I helped her up and brought her inside. I thought maybe if she just sat inside until I closed, I could get her home safely.

She didn't say anything, just some groaning sounds. Her eyes were glassy and her breath left no doubts about what she'd been drinking. She smelled like a beer keg had spilled all over her.

"Oaaaahhhh. Errrrrrrrrrrrrrrrgggglll."

163

I had to do some announcing and when I came back she had relocated herself to the manager's office and had heaved on the carpet. Great timing, Amy.

I did my best to clean it up, but I did a sorry job of it. Little brown paper towels, all I could find, did little for the stain or the smell. I was sure it was really going to stink like stale beer and vomit in the morning. When I closed the station I practically carried her to my car and drove her to her house. She moaned a few times in my car. But, at least she didn't lose her cookies again in my front seat.

All the lights were out. I rang the bell, a porch light came on. Her mother peered through a narrow window in the door and then opened it.

"What on earth…….?"

"She's had a tough night, and she really needs some sleep."

Her Mom grabbed her arm and pulled her sick limp body over her shoulder. I left as quickly as I could.

"Thank you," I heard her Mom say as her daughter started groaning. Probably had no idea what had been happening, or what she did for my boss's office carpet. I didn't need to explain to her all the night's details. I was just grateful to slip away from a very awkward moment.

As I drove home I figured I was going to have to face the music soon.

Not surprisingly, the next day I was asked not to come back to work. There had also been a story around school that I had given away a bunch of the station's records, which wasn't true. But, I could only say I didn't do it, and I didn't think I was very convincing. The discovery of the odor and the carpet stains vaulted me way over the top.

It was time to change course and let it go. It sure hurt to leave like that after four happy years. It was a good job. But, my future was pointed in another direction.

THE MIDDLE YEARS

20

JULY 16, 1967, I entered the United States Air Force. They flew me to San Antonio, Texas, Lackland Air Force Base, for six weeks of basic training and then on to Colorado Springs. It didn't take long before I started making an impression with my superiors.

We were marching down a quiet street at Lackland Air Force Base. It was a hot afternoon, way over 90 degrees, humid and sticky. A fly chose my nose, out of 300 or so men, all dressed alike in green fatigues. It flew right at my nose and started buzzing. Over and over it crashed into my face. Tolerating it only so long, I swiped at it with my hand, and my arm movements caught the eye of Master Sergeant Donnelly.

"You there. Fall out. What's your name?"

"Sir. My name is Stephen Knapp. Sir."

"Sir" was suddenly one of the most popular words there I'd ever seen. We had to use it where ever and when ever possible.

"Knapp. What in the hell do you think you're doin'?"

"I was swatting a fly, Sir."

"Well. Isn't that a fine how-do-you-do? Knapp, I'm going to make an example out of you, so that you will remember we don't swat flies. Is that clear?"

"Yes, sir. Thank you, sir."

"I want you to go back to C Barrack and ask if I'm there."

"Yes, sir," I looked him dubiously.

"Go on. Run!"

He was serious. I started to run.

"Stop! It's that way. Oh, my God. This kid's a real prize one, I'll tell ya. Probably doesn't even know which way's up. Where do they find these kids anyway?"

I had started in the wrong direction. I reversed and took off again, trying to ignore his comments.

After a three block run I knocked on the door and I asked the guard on duty if Master Sergeant Donnelly was there.

"No. He's out there marching down the street."

"Yeah. I know. He told me to ask you."

We both shrugged our shoulders and shook our heads and gave each other looks of complete disbelief in the logic of it all. I left him laughing under his breath and jogged back to the line.

"Knapp. Come here. Did you ask if I was in the basement?"

"No, Sir."

He and I both knew there was no basement. This was just a mind game.

"Well, run back and ask if I'm in the basement."

"Yes, Sir."

I repeated this exercise several more times inquiring about his presence in the attic, the patio, the swimming pool, and finally I was allowed to rejoin the group who had just completed marching exercises for the day. I had the pleasure of running 30 blocks in stifling heat with heavy boots on. None too soon for me we were moved on to Colorado.

I wondered if I would be able to predict the weather like I did at home. I wondered if I was going to fit in with this military stuff. It was all so different. I could tell just looking around I had never been in a place even remotely similar to this one. It wasn't just the mountains and the buildings. It was the way everyone walked and talked and acted.

The setting was beautiful. Huge rugged mountains and a multi-spired chapel so big it dominated the campus. I'd never been in the mountains before but they looked like they were so close I could reach out a touch them. I was enamored and found myself just staring at them. Having looked at flat Kansas horizons all my life I wasn't at all prepared for this incredible view.

My first room-mate, Fred, had been in the Air Force for two years before coming here. Fred was already a veteran. He knew all the tricks.

"You don't want to crawl under your covers at night. You sleep on top of your bed and don't wrinkle the covers. Watch." He crawled under my bed and pulled the side covers down and under. "Now watch me do this." He took a safety pin and pinned the under sides of the sheets together. Then he pinned the blanket together in the same way.

"Now this bed is tight." He flipped a quarter in the air and it bounced. "OK. You pass. Keep it this way and you won't have to spend twenty minutes each morning making your bed."

"How do you sleep?" I asked him. "Seems like the only way is to lie so still you don't move."

"You got it. Wear your sweats to stay warm. In a few nights you'll have it mastered. You'll sleep motionless."

"This is crazy, you know?"

"Yeah. Well. I don't think about that. I just do it."

"Fred. This is exactly what I don't need, but I'll try it."

My habit of falling asleep at unpredictable times began in my senior year of high school. It had followed me from Coffeyville, to Colorado, only worse. Maybe it was studying over three hours every night. Maybe it was getting up at 5:30 am and running five miles every morning up and down mountain trails before breakfast. Maybe it was some other reason.

Maybe something was wrong with me. Nobody else there did it but me.

I would fall asleep in class almost daily, but never during the same time period. This caused me problems with teachers who started issuing me demerits which was bad because they cost points against my whole squadron. This enraged Master Sergeant Entwhistle, who was in charge of every move we made.

He came in my room one morning at 5 am. Knapp, "Get out of that bed now!" He kicked my waste basket across the room, strewing cigarette ashes, and bits of papers randomly about the room.

Master Sergeant Entwistle was a seasoned career veteran. He'd been a lot of places over the years, served a lot of different tour of duties and this was his bread and butter until retirement, only a few years away. No young kid named Stephen Knapp was going to ruin anything for him. He could be as tough as we needed to be to keep things in line. I didn't have a chance.

"I'm so pissed at you. My whole squadron is pissed at you. You are about as stupid a monkey trying to make love to a football."

He slapped his hand down on my desk hard enough it would have crushed anything underneath it.

"Here's what you are going to do this weekend. No fun and games for you, you idiot. You will report to the security guard at the front gate, in full blue dress uniform, every hour on the hour, from 1800 hours on Friday until 0600 hours on Monday morning. And you will not miss or be late to a one of them. I want to see your signature on every hour. You got all that? Is that perfectly clear?" he screamed at me.

"Yes, Sir."

"And you will learn not to fall asleep ever again. You got that? Huh. You got that, Knapp?"

"Yes, sir." What else could I say?

He stomped out of my room, sidestepping the mess he had made. He looked back at me in his usual arrogant fashion. "I'll get you if you don't. You'll pay. Big time."

This may have been among the craziest things I had ever done, but I did it to try and avoid whatever he had thought up that would have been even worse. I dressed up in full uniform, shiny shoes, neck tie tied, the whole nine yards, and I walked 15 minutes to the front gate, signed in, and the guard noted the time. I saluted him and turned around to go back to my room, which took me another 15 minutes. I hade 15 minutes to undress, rest, dress again, and begin the cycle again. A few times I skipped a few steps and just tried to sleep a few minutes sitting in a chair without getting undressed.

From Friday night, all day Saturday, all day Sunday through Monday early morning I followed this inane routine, one hour at a time. I became more tired and more exhausted with each ensuing hour. There was no time to eat a real meal, no time to study, no time to watch a TV program.

And, to no one's surprise who knew what I was going through, on Monday morning in my first class within moments of sitting at my desk I fell soundly asleep.

A few classes later I fell asleep standing at the blackboard halfway into a calculus problem. There were three sets of nice numbers that I had written in chalk, then my hand dropped down, dragging the white chalk in a straight line to the bottom of the board, and my sleeve got lots of chalk dust on it as I stood there, asleep, oblivious to everything that was going on.

Smitty woke me up. "Hey. Knapp. Snap to." He dug his fist into my rib just hard enough I felt it. "Class is over. Go to your next class. You got five minutes."

Smitty was a friend. I only had as few of them. He was one. He was an Air Force brat. Lived all over the world with his Dad on air force bases. We got along great. He didn't have many friends either. Not close ones.

He was egregiously overweight, which caused him all kinds of problems, until we had wrestling. His weight gave him a huge edge during the competition. But, all the running we did daily was hard on him.

The next day we had to take a special class on the other side of the campus and we got on board a bus to get there. I fell asleep standing on the bus and was left there still asleep when everyone else got off. The bus driver had to shake me or I would've missed the class.

My sleeping now has raised a few eyebrows and somehow I was shuffled into the school's psychiatrist. I felt a sense of safety there because I was granted patient immunity. His office was like a completely different world. I was free there. I could say anything without fear of reprisal or discipline. We talked about my childhood. My parents. My golf game. Lots of things.

He told me he was Dr. Timothy Leary's (famed user of LSD) room mate in college. After four visits with no conclusions I was scheduled for medical tests.

"Mr. Knapp. There's obviously something unusual going on here. Your sleep behavior is not normal. We know you can't control it. We need to run some tests on you. I want you to be back here at 0800 hours tomorrow."

The EEG, electro encephalograph, was amazing. A brilliant piece of medical equipment. That's for sure. Two nurses stuck about 50 needles attached to wires into my head at different places. The wires all flowed into a machine which drew graphs.

"Ouch! Ouch!" Each anode stuck me like a needle as she punctured my skin. "Is this necessary?"

"I'm afraid so. Just a few more here. It's not that bad."

"Thanks." I didn't need someone else to tell me what hurt and what didn't. It----flat----hurt. E—v—e—r-y - time.

I didn't say that out loud, but my wincing with each prick had to have let them know this was no picnic for me.

"OK. Mr. Knapp. We're done here for a while. Just lie there still and go to sleep so we can measure what happens when you are in a sleep mode."

"Yes ma'am."

ARE YOU KIDDING ME? I was in so much pain with 50 needles stuck in my head there was no way of falling asleep. Absolutely impossible. Who dreamed that one up I'll never know, but I'll bet they never had it done to themselves. I just laid there in pain and hoped it would end soon.

The next day I went back to the psychiatrist. He told me I had narcolepsy, but not ordinary narcolepsy. "Narcolepsy is a sleeping disorder, the symptom is an uncontrollable propensity to sleep."

"You see, Mr. Knapp, narcolepsy is usually accompanied by certain organic chemical imbalances in the brain. Test results show no such imbalances. Very curious. Never seen anything like it."

"However, you do need some help. I'm going to give you a prescription, a drug called Dexedrine. This should help you stay awake. If it doesn't just let me know, But, I think you'll see a big difference."

Boy, did I.

Life, as I knew it, started changing immediately, and for the better. I was alert in class. My grades began to improve. I wrote an English paper on descriptive word uses where I scored second highest out of the 300 plus men taking that class.

And, my physical performance was enhanced unbelievably. We had a competition similar to an Olympic marathon. There are ten activities – running, jumping, throwing, swimming – and points were awarded on a scale depending on how fast, or how far, or whatever for that event. I finished 19th overall! I was competing with all three squadrons of first class level. This included the football team, the basket ball team, the track team, the gymnastics team, the wrestling team and just a bunch of bigger, taller, stronger, very physically fit young men who had to meet the same certain physical requirements as a part of their admission and they exercised rigorously every day. I was not a giant at 5' 8", 145 pounds, so finishing 19th out over 300 athletes all in superb condition was unbelievable.

Master Sergeant Entwhistle backed off. He even complimented me once. "Hey, Knapp. You seem to be coming around, huh?" He smiled and his eyes went halfway up his forehead. "Maybe I was wrong about you."

It was right after that I had a conversation with Captain Mark Phillips. I bet him I could swim two lengths of the school's Olympics sized pool underwater with no breaths after I was in the water. I did it. He didn't want to pay me the pack of cigarettes I had won, but Sgt. Entwistle backed me and made him pay me. The Captain didn't smoke and deplored anyone who did.

That was a compliment coming from him. Believe me.

I became friends with my new room-mate John Jones. John and I hit it off day one. He taught me the "gotcha game."

We were sitting together at lunch facing opposite directions and he said, "Oh my God, there's your mother." Naturally, I turned around to look at …… nothing. Obviously, she wasn't there. She was in Kansas.

"Gotcha."

This was a game we played often, trying to catch each other off guard and bite at something unbelievable or so foolish you felt stupid after it was too late. I was a fast learner and I didn't like looking naive. He didn't get me too many more times after that, and I got him a few myself in return.

John Jones was the most amazing beer drinker I had ever seen. On a typical Saturday night we would walk into a bar in Denver and he would make an offer at the first table with guys sitting around that he could chug a glass of beer faster than anyone at that table. There was usually a taker and John quickly reviewed the rules.

"You start with a full glass, held to your lips and somebody says go, the first to put the empty glass on the table wins a pitcher from the loser." John never lost.

He threw the beer toward the back of his throat without swallowing and the glass came down completely empty in about a second. The other guy was still swallowing his last sip.

"Go!"

John tossed the glass back and hit the table.

"Hey, bartender, need another pitcher over here."

We never paid for beer. I saw him pour a whole pitcher down his throat once. He never gulped or swallowed or caught a breath or anything. Amazing. Truly amazing.

John introduced me to Doug, a high school friend of his, one night. John took out an old girl friend and Doug took me out and introduced me to marijuana. I only did it a few times, but it was definitely a different feeling. I was scared of getting caught and I gave it up after that.

I believed for the first time that this would all work out. I was going to survive. I was going to eventually graduate. I was really going to be a pilot, just like the commercial pilot on the American Airlines plane I met when I was 10. It was going to be a great life. Not just OK. It was going to be great – "fabulous" as Mom would say. Dad would be extremely proud of his son for the first time in a long time. He was an officer in the Navy. It would be fitting that I became an officer in the Air Force.

That's why he helped me get the appointment, or maybe it just was a free education.

Even before Christmas I had called home telling Dad I wanted to quit and come home. He talked me into staying and gutting it out. Now it would be worth it. I'm glad I stayed. I had proven a lot to myself and everyone else around me. It was all going to work out.

Then they pulled the Dexedrine. I tried to get a refill because I was out and it was denied.

"No more refills, Mr. Knapp, the pharmacist said to me "the doctor made a point to mention it about you. You're on your own." There was no mistake. Officials at the Academy wanted to see how I would respond without it. How would I act drug free?

The next day I fell asleep in my first class.

If there was a God who was engineering this life of mine, He must have changed His mind, or just decided to redirect my life's course. Or maybe, this was a set of experiences that would somehow enhance my life at some future time. Maybe there was something to be gained here that I was just missing the point at that moment and it would be crystal clear eventually. Maybe this was just a dirty trick played on me. Maybe it was Karma. Maybe I had some crazy disease and I didn't know it. Fat chance of that.

I was told I couldn't be on drugs and be in the Air Force. I was medically discharged. They invented a disorder just for me. Inorganic narcolepsy. There is no such thing in the medical books, but that's what they said I had. That's what it would say in my files.

No more dreams of being a pilot. No more Air Force Academy. No more great life. No future squat.

John hadn't heard the news yet. I was told to immediately stop attending class and went back to sleep in my room mid-day. John walked in and saw me under the covers.

"Steve. Is that you?"

"No. I'm just a guy who looks and sounds like Steve lying in his bed."

That was my last time playing "gotcha" with John. He broke his arm playing football a few days later and I never saw him again after that. I moved to my own room and after full clearance I went back to Kansas.

No more military, ever again. I got a draft notice for the army soon after I arrived home. But, having gone 99% of the way through the process without a problem they told me "if the Air Force doesn't want you, the Army doesn't want you, either." I was classified 4-Y, and a career in the military was now completely out of the picture forever.

The one positive thread that came out of that year's horrendous experience was that I did get a chance to play a round of golf with the Air Force Academy golf coach, Capt. Shot Davis, before I left. I hadn't even hit a ball since I flew to Lackland months ago, but I shot a respectable 2 over par. After our round he said he could get me a golf scholarship at Utah State University, in Logan, Utah, because of his connections there. Having nothing else in the works, and had not tried to get anything going, I accepted that offer. I contacted the coach at Utah State a few days after I was rejected by the Army.

Utah was further away from Kansas than Colorado and I still wanted to keep all the distance I could get from my dysfunctional family. A month later I was on my way to Utah.

21

I WAS SURE Mom and Dad were embarrassed I didn't last at the Academy. We never talked about it, but I knew they were disappointed in me. I had received an offer to go to Kansas State University and play on their golf team, but they didn't offer scholarships for golf. Utah State offered a some assistance, so that's where I went. I didn't bother to look anywhere else.

I figured I was mostly on my own financially. I needed transportation. A car. A used car. A cheap used car. Tim Sage's grandmother had one for sale. Tim and I played a lot of pool when I was in high school. Her 1953 Dodge Coronet, only had 52,000 miles on it and it had a Hemme engine. I didn't know what that was, but, I guessed it was OK. Tim said it was a good thing to have.

I bought it for $75. I put two good used tires for $40 on the front to replace the bald ones. The radio didn't work. I could not possibly travel across the country to Utah without a radio. I bought a new RCA radio that ran on 8 D batteries. The radio and batteries were $50.

I was set. Suitcase, golf clubs, my Ampax reel to reel tape player and everything I needed to live there was packed in the trunk with plenty of room left over.

Logan, Utah, greeted me with beautiful mountains, similar to Colorado, but with more snow on the tops. The big difference was my freedom. No more mandatory 3 ½ hours studying in my room every night. No more getting up at 5:00 am to go run five miles on mountain paths. No more Master Sgt. Entwhistle yelling in my face. And I was going to get to play golf. Lots of golf. Time for practice, time for whatever I wanted.

The first small town in Utah I came to had a nice little restaurant and I was getting hungry after the sixteen hours drive through Kansas and Colorado. I ordered after waiting to be seated and they were busy so I could see it would a while before I was served. I pulled out a deck of cards and started playing solitaire.

"We don't allow gambling in here. Could you please put those away?" I looked up on disbelief at the manager.

"Sure." I complied. I thought to myself, this isn't gambling. You can't gamble with yourself. *If you want to see gambling…,* but I didn't say anything.

I wondered if Utah and I would get along together.

Enrollment was enough to make me want to crawl in a hole and die.

"Name please. Last name. K? Stand in this line." I stood in that line for four hours.

"We don't have your name listed. Stand in this line over there."

I stood in that line over there for another four hours.

"No. We don't have you listed. Did you fill out enrollment papers for admission?""

"Yes."

"Well. We don't have them. No forms, no doctor's shot records. You will have to start all over again. Please stand in this line. Uh, it's too late today. Come back tomorrow."

Next day wasn't any better.

"Well, why don't we have your enrollment papers? What's wrong with you? You haven't paid anything. Who's your advisor? Don't have one yet? You don't have any of the right forms. Go stand in this line, no, never mind. Go to Dr. Samulson's office. Grayson Building on the other side of the courtyard."

"Sorry. Can't help you. You need an advisor before I can help you. Go back over there and stand in the line over at admissions."

And, on and on it went for three days. I was still not enrolled. I'd stood in every line imaginable. No school, no golf team, no scholarship. No enrollment. No class schedule. No major. No advisor. I was a non-person. My college career was looking very bleak.

I was a complete unknown – "Like a Rolling Stone" – Bob Dylan. I thought about going back to Kansas and see in they would still take me at K. State.

Finally,…."Ah. Hah. Here it is. It's all here. Look. You filled it out with an "H." We can't read your writing. It looks like "Hnapp." It was filed under the "H's". "That's why no one could find you. Let's make this a "K" and now we can get you started. Go stand over there." She was right. It did look like an "H".

I adapted quickly to college life once I got on board. Mostly. I had a 7:30 am Basic Algebra class, but after that it was a breeze. I took 15 hours, five 3-hour classes, and I was off campus by noon so I could play and practice golf every afternoon with the team. My game came back and was better than ever. My grades were so-so, but I was absorbing so many new things. I told everyone my major was golf, and my minor was life.

Everybody was from somewhere else, San Diego California, Newark, New Jersey, Scarsdale, New York, and a few were from Utah. It was interesting to get to know so many new people. I learned about Mormonism – it was ubiquitous. I learned how to drink coffee and stay up very late talking to my new friends. I reacquainted myself with popular music because everybody listened to it in the dorms. Music was not heard very often at the Academy. The Moody Blues became my favorite group.

There wasn't much golf to be played for me until spring. This fact became quite apparent to me after our first snow. Then the next week more snow. Then the next week more snow. And more and more. It never melted. This wasn't Kansas where I played many fall and winter days. Even in Colorado the snow disappeared after a warm spell. There were no warm spells there. Every morning I woke up and went crunch, crunch as my tennis shoes squashed the newly fallen snow.

Smiling at me as I listened to him in disbelief one evening, a guy name Joe told me it snowed about 500 inches a year, and I wouldn't see the ground until mid-March. I thought, "Why did I come here if I couldn't play golf but six months out of the year?" Well, it was definitely a little late for that now. Very definitely not well thought out.

A couple of new friends, Dave and Gary, that I had met in Algebra class asked me to a party in Salt Lake City one Saturday night. "Sure," I said. They gave me excellent directions. Getting there was no problem. The return trip would be a different story.

I drank a good amount of beer and met a lot of new people, mostly from Salt Lake City, 80 miles from where I was going to school, and it was not likely I would be making that trip on a regular basis. Then again, maybe so.

"Hi. I'm Pam."

Pam was beautiful, very friendly, and slightly drunk. We talked for a few hours and had a good time getting to know about each other, and then we went downstairs and found a quiet place to make out for a while. That was all. It was late and I had to get back. I politely said goodbye to Pam reluctantly and left the party still going strong..

I walked outside and it was eerie. The night sky was totally black, no stars, no lights, or no moon. There was a haze hanging over the earth like a foggy canopy and I was just underneath it. The snow was falling in large soft flakes and my car was not recognizable. I found it only because I had parked illegally and was close to a stop sign down at the end of the street from the party.

It was an incredibly silent world I found myself walking in and I was amazed how still it was. I had to brush off all the snow on the front and rear windshields. It was like heavy white dust, sticking together in clumps. I had to check the directions I had left in the front seat earlier that evening. I had no idea where I was. Nothing looked familiar. Somehow I made my way to State Roads 89-91 to get on the road out of town, and then the fun really started.

The din of the city light did provide a little bit of help, seeing signs every so often. I was comfortable that I was going the right way. As I got out into the more rural edges of Salt Lake signs became fewer and fewer. I looked at my watch – 2 am, it was at least two hours or more to get back to Logan. It started to snow heavier.

My windshield wipers couldn't keep up with the falling snow. I couldn't see out of the rear windshield at all and the wipers started to go under the mass of snow on the front windshield. The wipers slid back and forth but the glob of snow didn't move and I couldn't see too well. I pulled over, got out and wiped all the snow off both front and back windows and climbed back in.

I could no longer discern the pavement and the lanes of the highway. There was just snow in front of me and behind me, and darkness overhead. The snow seemed to just appear, coming from out of the darkness further up.

I could pull over and sit in the car until daylight, but I might be buried in snow by then, or run out of gas and freeze to death. The tank was showing ¼ full. Not a good amount for staying there. I looked a second time at the dark road ahead and saw a faint line of tire tracks, one set of treads, one thin impression that the snow had not quite filled in yet. That had to be my ticket back.

I followed the tracks. After a good hour, the snow fall slowed and I could see tail lights bobbing up and down ahead of me. When it went over a hill I lost it, then it would reappear while I was level with it again. He was leading me. Completely. I was driving on utter faith that his driving was taking me safely home to Logan.

I wondered if he knew I was following him. I wonder if it's a he or a she driving. I wondered, whoever it was, if they knew where they were going. I said a prayer that he or she or they would get home safely. It was a very safe bet if he or she or they didn't make it, neither would I. I wondered if anyone knew that my life was counting on those tracks. I doubted it.

"Nights in White Satin"…the words flowed as I sang out loud to myself to keep myself awake. It was after 4 am and I had no idea how much farther I had to go. I kept going, thinking I was going to make it. Believing the tracks were my only hope to survive that night. I had to keep going.

Mile after mile there was no point of reference other than the tire marks. No billboards. No trees. No road signs. Not even reflectors, or illuminated lane markings.

It was snow and darkness and tread marks. And, once in a while, bobbing red tail lights, playing hide and seek with my life in the balance. My gas gauge was inching perilously closer to E.

When the sign welcoming me to the city if Logan came into view I breathed a heavy sigh. "Thank you, Lord," and "Thank you, also" to whoever bravely put tire tracks out there for me to follow safely to my destination. I never got close enough to ever know who he, or she or they were. But, if I ever got the chance, I would thank them greatly.

The cold temperatures outside made one appreciate hot showers, and I discovered that our dorm showers were able to get quite hot. So hot it would sting the skin. I liked that for some strange reason, and turned the showers on as hot as I could make them. If I withstood the hottest temperatures long enough, it would actually feel freezing. It was weird, I know, but I did it a few times.

My skin would be red for quite a while after I got out. And in about 3 three days I would itch across my back side. It took a few times before it dawned on me I had burned my skin in the shower and the dry itching was my skin peeling off. The itching wasn't worth the thrill of feeling freezing hot water in the shower, so I gave it up after a few times.

Jack was a guy on my dorm floor that I didn't know very well, but he asked me if I wanted to go to a party with him.

"Sure." I went along. Actually, I drove which was why he asked me, I think. We coasted into a parking place close to the house and walked in. I didn't know anyone there.

It wasn't a very big place, but people were sitting anywhere there was room. Music droned lightly, many conversations were taking place in small groups.

"Hi. Wanta beer? In the refridge." She leaned her head to the side and giggled. "I'm Angie."

'Why don't you show me where it is? I'm Steve."

"Follow me."

The kitchen was empty and we sat down at the small table with two blue slightly stained chairs. Nothing fancy about the apartment. It was cold.

"Is your heater broke? It's a little frosty in here you know?"

"Well. We dress for it. You aren't from around here are you? You look like you're ready to go to a spring picnic."

No wonder. I looked at myself. Golf shirt, light sweater, wind breaker, jeans, tennis shoes. "What's wrong with that?" I thought.

"Nope. Kansas. Quite a different climate. Most definitely. Never been to Utah before. I mean like growing up or anything. I'm a Midwesterner. Born and raised in Kansas."

Angie was stocky with a round face, freckles, long brownish auburn hair, and a big smile. Everything she said had a little needle in it. And she laughed a lot. "So you are like Toto, huh. Wizard of Oz, you know? She giggled."

"Look. There is really a lot more to Kansas that the impression one gets from the movie. I'd like to show you the vast fields of wheat, the beautiful rolling hills, and grassy plains. You should see the fields of wheat or corn that stretch for miles like they have no end. And all the people are great. Real friendly. Easy to get to know. Real down to earth kind of people."

"I'd like that. I'm from Wyoming. Big Piney. Ever heard of it?" Her eyes kept studying me. Not sure to believe me. Not sure to trust me. "It's right in the middle of a lot of sage brush. Nothing pretty around there at all. Biggest town around is Kemmerer. You've probably never of that either, huh? Of course, we do have mountains, and Yellowstone National Park. Got any mountains in Kansas?" She knew the answer, but she wanted to dig at me.

"Nope. Sounds like you grew up in a small town. I grew up in a small town, too. We may have some similar stories about that. Everybody in your town know everybody else? Gossip runs freely faster than the wind?"

"Oh. Yeah. Let's have that beer and keep talking."

I was playing with the pop top, but hadn't opened it.

We sat there and talked until the crowd left. We covered a myriad of subjects, how we grew up, where we went on vacations, what we liked to do for fun, what music we liked. We had absolutely nothing in common from growing up as far as interests or experiences, but it was enjoyable talking and exploring each other's background. We did both smoke Marlboros and drink Budweiser, beyond that we were as far apart as two people could be.

She wasn't athletic. She wasn't very popular as far as dating. She only liked country western music. She hadn't traveled out of the state of Wyoming very far. She didn't have the bigger picture awareness I had about the world. My trips and experiences in Michigan, Indianapolis, Mexico, Colorado, Texas, Oklahoma, Iowa, Missouri, Illinois, and Florida, as well as Kansas, had given me a much wider perspective. So, I thought, anyway. One thing we did have in common was laughter. We amused each other frequently which lead to trading one funny story to the next.

I guess Jack caught a ride with someone else. I noticed it got quiet in the other room.

"I think I'd better get going. Thanks for the beer." I headed for the door. I looked around. Everyone else had left.

"Nice talking with you. See ya."

"Bye," she said, smiling.

I went out to my car. Put my key in and Rrrererererer. Rrererererer. Great. It wouldn't start. Guess what? Outta gas. Past E. How'd that happen? How stupid was that?

Barely made it back from Salt Lake City and forgot to fill up. Perfect timing, coldest night of my life and I was stuck there in a strange area of town with no way to drive back to the dorm. Definitely, too far to walk. Jeeeeez.

Embarrassed I went back to the front door. Finding heat was a greater motivator than not swallowing my pride. I was already shivering from just being in their cold apartment for three hours. The lights were already out inside. I wasn't looking forward to what I had to ask.

Knock. Knock.

"Who's there?" It was Angie's voice.

"It's me. Steve. I feel stupid but I need to ask a favor. I'm out of gas. Could you take me to a gas station?"

She opened the door. She laughed. "You're kidding? Right?" Then she cocked her head. "Do you run out of gas a lot? What? They have gas stations all over the place, every other corner in Kansas? No need to plan ahead. Right?" Clearly, the thought of going out driving me around as fresh snow was falling did not excite her at all.

"You know it's about 10 below right now. And it's snowing. The nearest gas station is closed. I don't know where the next one is. Ya see I go there before I run out, during the day so I don't have to search for one this time of night. Besides that, I've had my share of beer tonight."

She looked my car. Under the snow she could see my old Dodge Coronet, 1953 model. "Is that what you are driving? No wonder you ran out of gas. It probably all leaked out. How you could drive something that old? I can see you'll never be accused of being one of those high octane testosterone type drivers. Huh? Hah. How many weeks did it take you to drive here from Kansas anyway? Pony express could've gotten here faster, I'll bet"

She was really giving to me.

"Thanks. When you're done with all of that, can you please just take me? There's got to be something open out there. I'm going to die if I have to walk. I might turn into a snowman just standing here talking to you. What do you say?"

"I got a better idea. Stay here tonight. I'll take you in the morning."

"Errrr. You sure? OK. Deal."

I had no feeling in my toes as we climbed up the steps that lead to her door. Crunch. Crunch. The snow had a way of letting you know its going to make you feel as cold as you possibly could feel. This was it, too. I was there. It couldn't feel colder. She opened the door for me.

"After you." I held the door for her.

"Thanks."

I walked right behind her.

"If you sleep out here," she motioned to the couch in the living room," you'll freeze to death. I've got an electric floor heater in my bedroom. Follow me."

She didn't turn the lights on. I stepped behind her slowly, trusting she was taking me somewhere warmer. I prayed it was warmer. I was shivering all over and my teeth were chattering, and my toes felt painfully numb, like someone had just hit them with a dull sledge hammer.

We walked into her bed room. It was small. A double bed and a chest of drawers was all I could see.

"You take the left side I take the right side. Keep to your side. Keep your hands by your sides. Don't try anything. You wouldn't want to anyway. It's my time of the month."

I did not have the willingness to volunteer that I was still a virgin. I was terribly ignorant about sex. It had never been discussed in my house growing up. Somehow it never came up on the fairways of Coffeyville Country Club. I didn't know squat about sex. She never knew how safe she was. Her virtue was more secure than all the gold at Fort Knox. Her electric floor heater glowed an orange brilliance in the corner by the bed and I started getting warmer. That's all I wanted.

As my teeth chattered I muttered, "I'm very grateful you let me stay here. Thank you. You didn't have to. You didn't have to even answer the door."

"Yeah, I did. I knew it was you."

After we got gas the next morning she asked me over for dinner. I accepted. She cooked venison and potato pancakes. Delicious, and completely new to me. Both of them.

"They don't have these foods in Kansas?"

"No. Not that I know about any way. And, by the way, just curious, do you make a habit of sharing your bed with strangers you just met?"

"Not hardly. Only guys from Kansas who don't have enough sense to fill up their tank which causes them to run out of gas. And even then, only so they won't freeze to death." She always had a cocky look about her when she dug into me like that. Her eyes squinted, head cocked and the corners of her mouth became more sharply pronounced.

Nice comeback.

Whatever I threw at her, she threw it right back, sometimes one better than mine.

"Ok. Ok. I'll lay off. You saved me. Thank you. I admit it. Got any more beer?" We both laughed.

We started seeing each other every few evenings or so for the next several months. We studied together. We ate together. We drank coffee at the student union together.

"Hey. Smart guy." She called me on the phone about 9 o'clock on a Wednesday night.

"Yeah, what?"

"I need your help on some homework." This was reasonable. I'd helped her before. She was a Psychology major and we even had one class together.

"Be right there." She had moved to a nicer apartment with three roommates much closer to campus.

But, when I get to her place she didn't want my help. She wanted me. It was awkward. I was clumsy. But, it was a wonderful night.

I got up the next morning to go to the bathroom to relieve myself.

"Where's the restroom?"

"Second door on the left," she directed nonchalantly with one arm in the air, finger pointing parallel to the floor.

Neither Angie nor I knew at that moment that her room-mate, Diane, was just stepping out of the shower. When we met face to face at the bathroom door she was completely naked, unprepared with any thought there was a guy entering the bathroom from the other side.

"Aaaaaaaaaaaaaaaayyyyyyyyyyyyyy! Get out of here!"

She quickly covered her chest with one arm and her crotch with the other, and I did an about face fast enough not to notice anything. But, it was a point of contention between the two girls for quite some time.

When I returned to Angie's bedroom we both laughed uproariously. It was just one of those things.

Life was good, different, much different than at the Academy, and I had so much freedom. If I really wanted to skip a class and sleep in, I could and no one yelled at me. They didn't even take notice. In a few months time my sleeping in class propensities stopped and never returned. I became about as normal a guy as I had been in a long time.

I was the low scorer in many of the golf matches we played that first year and as the spring semester ended we had an athlete's banquet. Football and basketball players were there as well as the less important sports like golf. I was honored with a silver engraved plate for being the best golf player for that year at Utah State University. I was very proud of that plate, but someone in my dorm room dropped it two days later and put a 6 inch dent in it.

My glory was short-lived. A few days later I received a report I had been put on academic suspension. I had not given my finals a very serious effort, and I even skipped one because I figured I could take the class again and do better. Since I had only recently discovered the powers of coffee, I thought could simply drink lots of it and stay up all night studying. I drank tons of coffee, stayed up four days and four nights straight during finals. As I took my last exam things started flying around in front of me. I was hallucinating. This was a first for me and it frightened me.

The news got worse as the golf coach, Dean Candland, the same guy who praised me and handed me the silver plate at the dinner, told me I was off the team until I raised my grades.

"No. Please." I pleaded. "I'll do better. I'll study harder. I promise."

He was firm. "Get your grades up first. Then we'll talk about you getting back on the team."

Hello summer school, here I come.

This was a key turning point for me. I had been a Journalism major, but there was only one journalism professor who taught all the journalism classes and I couldn't stand him. There was only one way to write – his way. We disagreed philosophically on how to write and he definitely had the upper hand, so I was never going to see things his way and I bolted.

Of all the classes I had taken Psychology was the subject I seemed to have the most interest in and in which I had made the best grades. So, I changed my major to Psychology and a year later added Sociology as a double major.

It was absolutely crucial I made two A's in the summer courses. I needed two A's to get my GPA back to where I could be considered to be removed from academic suspension which would clear me to be back on the golf team again.

I knew I could do this, but added pressure came unexpectedly.

"Students, this is a short course and so we are going to be able to just take one final exam. What you make on that will be what you get for a grade for the course." Early Child Psychology was not a difficult subject, but putting all the marbles in one bag made me very uncomfortable.

I attended every class. I took copious notes. I read psychology every night. I began to see the pages in my sleep.

Which actually helped me.

On the exam was a question, multiple choice answers, and two of the answers were so close to being the right one I had to stop and think twice, then three times. I closed my eyes. I began to mentally read the book page by page. I knew that answer. It was on the right side of the page. Second paragraph. Second sentence. I could see it in my mind. I read it again on the page. The answer was there. My photographic memory was clear as crystal.

Two other times on the test similar situations required that questions needed to be answered in the same way. Best of all, my memory worked! I made a 98%! I made the A I needed. The other class was easier and I made an A there, as well. By fall I had been reinstated to the school's golf team and regained the confidence of my golf coach.

Even though I made two A's that summer and was invited to rejoin the golf team, I never was again recognized at year end as the number one player on the team. I devoted more time to studies, and less time to golf. In the next three years I planned to take enough courses to graduate on time and another chapter of my life would end after graduation. I was determined to make that plan stick.

The great boxer Cassius Clay, now known as Muhammed Ali, was not boxing at the time in his career when I was at Utah State. As a conscientious objector with religious justification he avoided the draft, and went on a country wide campus tour speaking about his views.

I had to get some slacks dry cleaned for an upcoming golf tournament. The only dry cleaner I ever used was only a few blocks from campus. I walked toward the store's doorway with my wrinkled slacks hung over my shoulder. I moved into the doorway just as Ali was coming out and I blocked his way. He looked straight into my eyes.

"How's my man?" he said, and offered his hand with a big smile. I shook it.

"Pleased to meet you," I said, gawking at him with mouth wide open.

He winked and walked off to a limousine carrying a tuxedo that he had picked up there. Probably wore it that night.

I missed his presentation. I would have enjoyed it, but I was that committed to studying.

I started to drive home for Christmas, but I never made it out of town. My car had serious engine problems and I couldn't wait for major repairs. I flew as far as my money would take me which was Kansas City. A girl I knew there, whom I had met in high school at a Key Club convention, picked me up and took me to the bus station and by 4 am I was home. A week later I took a bus back to Utah and caught the Hong Kong flu somewhere along the way. I was in bed a week wanting to die I felt so horrible. That was as sick as I had ever been. Sickness in general was a rarity for me.

Dorm life had its limitations. My bedroom, which I shared with another Steve who was also on the golf team, was on the 7th floor of a large tall structure on campus.

Elevators were always so, and stairs were a hassle to walk up that far.

One of the things that annoyed me most was how the guy at the front desk could buzz my room through the PA system at any time, night or day, and say something stupid like "Is George Smith there? He has a visitor downstairs."

"Oh, sorry, wrong room. Well, if you see George tell him he has a guest here." This was very disruptive for sleeping, studying, or listening to the Moody Blues play "Nights in White Satin," my favorite song. It was just happening too often.

One night as a prank I snuck into the desk area about 3 am when it was unattended and put duct tape on all the buttons so all rooms would be called at once with a buzzing noisy alert. It didn't last for very long, but it felt good to do it. There were tons of complaints and somebody got in trouble, but not me.

I had a great friend in the dorm named Dick. We spent long hours just talking. It was wonderful to have someone to listen to me, and I listened to him and we both sounded more intelligent about the world. We also shared our inner thoughts and philosophies and seemed to always connect.

Early in the first semester his car, a Datsun, died and his Dad bought him a new one, except he had to go to Lake Tahoe to get it. This offered an opportunity for a terrific adventure. We skipped a week of school and hitch hiked all the way from Logan, Utah, to get his new car.

On the edge of town in Logan, we stood on the highway pointing our thumbs, looking hopeful someone would stop. Dick and I had packed the absolute minimal amount of supplies and clothing, all of which fit in a small backpack he carried. He had our thumbs out for only a few minutes when a car passed us, stopped, backed up to where we were and pulled down the window. Two girls squinted at us.

"Are you Rob and John? Uh, you're not you, are you?" They were momentarily bewildered, then embarrassment. They stopped to pick up two guys they knew, only we weren't those two guys. A case of mistaken identity. An uncomfortably awkward moment for them.

I broke the silence. "Sorry. This is Dick. I'm Steve." We smiled as earnestly as we possibly could.

"So, Dick and Steve, where you headed," one of them queried? They seemed nice enough to respond.

"Lake Tahoe, but if could get us to Salt Lake City that would help. Sorry we are not Rob and John, but we are two very nice guys." I smiled sheepishly. Salt Lake City was 80 miles away, but at least there was no snow. That would put us on a major highway and we could get lucky once we got there.

"Oh, I'm Jill. This is Sherry."

"Hi."

Dick and I looked at each other mentally crossing our fingers.

They whispered back and forth a few times. I guess we passed the visual litmus test.

"OK. We're going to Salt Lake and we have room so hop in."

We had a great time talking during the 80 mile drive through the mountains and when we stopped in Salt Lake to be let out they started whispering again. Then they went to a pay phone and called their homes. Minutes later they made a surprising offer.

"We have never been across the Utah-Nevada border and we've always wanted to. So, if you guys want, we can take you that far. There is a casino there and a few motels. We'll, Sherry and I, you know, we'll spend the night, and come back tomorrow morning. We've never gambled, never played a slot machine. I just want to see what its like, you know. We checked with our moms and talked them into it."

"Sounds like a deal we can't possibly match anywhere else. Drive on. Thanks so much"

We had fun shooting the breeze, telling stories about college, classes, teachers, all kinds of things. We laughed a lot, and never made a move to touch either of them.

I didn't ask them, but I figured they were Mormons, raised in the strict and protective Church's way of life, and hadn't seen much of the bigger world, very little of it, probably. It was a big adventure for them just to get out of town.

When we arrived it was getting dark. We said thanks and goodbye, and left them to check in at a motel, with no clue where we would stay.

"What do ya wanna do, Dick? Try and catch another ride or stay here?"

"I'm bushed. Let's get something to eat and think about it."

"Me, too. Sounds good."

We tossed down a hot dog and a beer. Then we ran into Jill and Sherry walking out of a small casino, and I convinced them if they let us sleep on the floor in their room, we promised to behave ourselves. They did and we did.

We all got some rest that night.

This was the epitome of a real "economy trip". So far Dick and I had traveled 80 miles, spent the night in a motel and spent $2 bucks each on dinner. We said thanks and goodbye to Jill and Sherry for the second time the next morning and made our way out to the edge of town.

It was already hot and it was only 8 am. Dick and I stood on the side of the highway and began the challenging task of getting someone to give us a lift. We weren't as lucky as we were with our two new friends we had waved goodbye to about an hour earlier.

Car after car whizzed by without stopping. A few acted like they didn't see us, but I know they did.

One man rolled down his window, slowed so we could hear him. "Hey. Get a car!"

Thanks a lot, buddy.

I could only stand there so long and I became so bored I pulled out Dick's Frisbee and crossed to the other side of the highway.

"Here you go, catch." We threw it back and forth in between cars for an hour until we got thirsty.

"I'm dying for some water, aren't you? Let's take a break" We had to go inside for a restroom break and find something to drink.

We resumed our position on the side of the road. We had not eaten anything since last night. The hot dog and beer had long since become only a memory. It was at least 110 degrees, no clouds, and not much breeze. The only time the air moved was when an 18 wheeler passed us by, but the quick surge of moving air was so hot and dry it was worse than just being still.

Not only was it was very dry and it was very dusty. Each car or semi that passed us stirred up a cloud of dust that coated our skin. I'm sure each breath I took sucked some particles of Nevada it into my lungs. I felt that hitch hiking had become not such a good idea.

Finally, somewhere around mid afternoon an old blue Carmen Ghia slowed and stopped by us off the road. A guy in a very French accent said, "Get in." It was tight, but it was the best offer we had had. It was the only offer we had had. We sat quietly and talked to Frenchman who had just made our day.

He was 25. Long hair and long beard. A hippie. Born in France but later moved to Quebec where he got a doctorate in something. It was noisy and I missed it, but I let him ramble on. He was drafted into their army. He said he was a French Canadian draft dodger. He fled to avoid incarceration. He was on his way to vanish and join a commune in southern California, but was in no particular hurry and no dead line. He offered to take us to Lake Tahoe, right to Dick's house. It was worth the half day baking in the sun to have him stop for us.

The Ghia made quite a rattling sound and hot air blew on my feet the whole way. The windows were down. No A/C. When I got out of his car, I fell forward. There was no feeling in my feet. I took off my shoes and socks and both feet were white with no color, no red or blue veins showing. No pink rosy red skin color. Just lily white. I guess the blowing heat and no circulation riding for eight hours in his car almost killed my feet. I rubbed them and slowly in about 20 minutes they came back to life. Then I could walk again.

Dick got his new car the next morning, and we went back to Utah. Nothing exciting happened on the way back. We must have had 5000 cars pass us by standing on the highway edge trying to appeal to anyone's kindness to pick us up. I guess thumbing a ride is more common in France. Maybe they just had more trust there, or fewer horror stories made the news. If we had been in Kansas, we would have been picked up in a heartbeat. Too bad it's not like that everywhere.

I looked up Sherry a few weeks later. We went out on a few dates. She mentioned she had a boyfriend who was in the army in Viet Nam. I didn't think our relationship was going to go very far, and I didn't want to get between him and her, so I stopped it. I started seeing Angie again.

A guy in a bar named Dave gave me a tablet one night. "Here. See you how you get off on this." I went back to the dorm and took it. He called it THC. Nothing happened. I waited for about 15 minutes and then I took a shower. Walking back to my room I lost consciousness.

The next thing I knew I was hearing music, "Magic Carpet Ride" by The Who. I was dancing to it, mentally. I was raising my head up and down to the beat of the song. I was in a stupor. The drug had kicked in all at once.

"Hey, Knapper, what are you doing? Are you OK?"

My head was in pain and blood was dripping down from my forehead. I wasn't fully aware of what I had just been doing. Consciousness came slowly. I was on the floor, on my knees, my head was bobbing up and down and I hit the floor with my head over and over to the beat of the music until I regained my thinking. I had blindly walked into the room three doors down from mine, no doubt drawn in by the stereo rock sounds. I was in a trance.

Jim Bailey told me it was totally bizarre. I came in without knocking. I got down on the floor on my knees and starting banging my head on the floor. He was sitting on his bed watching me in horror. It was the strangest thing he had ever seen. I believe him.

No more THC for me. Never again.

Another time Dick and I flew standby late at night to San Francisco for $20 each out of Salt Lake City. We spent the day walking from downtown to Seal's Point, around the coast over cliffs and back to where his friend's apartment was. We lived on two loaves of Fisherman's Wharf sour dough bread and had a blast the whole weekend. It was another great economy trip with wonderful lasting memories.

In most of our golf matches our team did not play well. We didn't have a great bunch of low scorers, but it was a terrific opportunity to play some very nice courses, for free. There were teams with better players and we always finished back in the pack.

As an example, BYU had Johnny Miller playing for them.

He's had a very successful career as a professional golfer, course designer and TV announcer. I played three rounds with him during the two years our college days overlapped. He was clearly on a different level than I was. He had greatness stamped all over him. My best round against him I shot 67. He shot 62.

We went to Las Vegas at spring break for a match with UNLV and the University of Arizona. We visited Caesar's Palace after the round. There with his band was Joe Frazier standing in the doorway next to a sign saying," Come See Joe Frazier and the Ding Dongs." I stood about 6 feet from him, but I did not get to shake his hand because he turned away abruptly and went up on a short stage. I had never seen a wider set of shoulders up close.

Strangely enough, in the course of just a couple of months I saw two world famous fighters – Ali and Frazier. That was always a good story over a few beers.

Angie and I became inseparable. For the next two years we went everywhere. We took trips to Wyoming, visited Jackson Hole. We went to Las Vegas once. We took several classes together. We even drove snow mobiles together at her family cabin.

"I think we should be engaged, don't you?" She asked me one day.

"Yeah, I guess so. Will you marry me?"

"Of course, dummy."

Mom had promised me a ring that belonged to her mother. Mom sent it to me after I called her. I gave it to Angie and we were officially engaged.

I got a letter from Janis. I was expecting a reaction to my announcement about Angie. We wrote every so often back and forth about college or people we knew from home, but this one was different.

"….Steve, I am sorry to hear of your grandmother's passing. My mother was talking to your mother earlier today and then my mother called me here in at KU….."

I was angry and hurt. It wasn't surprising my mother talked to her mother. It was a small town. The "grapevine" was faster than lightening. But, I didn't know my grandmother Weiss had died. Nobody bothered to tell me.

I called Mom but she said she didn't want to distract me and she wanted me to concentrate on school.

That did not help much. I was still hurt, but I was glad Janis had let me know. She was always thoughtful that way. If she could do anything to help she would do it. And we could always talk and make each other feel better.

Every Christmas, and summer, I came home for two weeks between semesters. I always spent time with Janis. She was dating around at KU, no one serious. It became almost expected we would spend time together when I came home. I had meals with her family as they had accepted me almost as another member of theirs. I always felt welcome there.

A typical meal at the Herman house was a feast. On the table was salad, Jell-O with fruit and marshmallows in it, rolls, home made banana bread, mashed potatoes and gravy, green beans, corn, and carved roast beef. Each was in its own container or dish and got passed around the table so everyone could choose what they wanted and how much. For desert there was always home made apple pie, or pumpkin pie served with ice cream on top. It was always scrumptiously delicious. Janis's mom, Dorothy, made it all. She was an amazing cook.

Janis was the oldest of five children and her mother and father both worked at the Yellow Front – a discount department store. It was only a few blocks from where their house was and one block from Holy Name Catholic Church where the Herman family walked every Sunday morning for mass. The Yellow Front was located one block from where my Dad and grandfather's offices, Knapp and Knapp Attorneys, were in downtown Coffeyville. My Dad and her father, Harry, attended high school together. I could stand in my grandfather's front yard and see Holy Name a half a block to the north on Spruce Street. I could hit a golf ball from Grandfather Knapp's house into Janis's back yard with a 8-iron. It was a small town. Everyone knew everything about everybody.

The elm trees in the Herman's front yard, like all the others in town that were among the once hundreds of bushy, tall, beautiful old trees, were dying from Dutch Elm disease. It was sad to see those giant pillars that lined both sides of all the major streets in town lose their leaves and become bare and lifeless. Of course, they looked like that every winter, but this was all year long. They were dead and had to be cut down. Most yards already had one or two large stumps sticking up a few inches above the ground where the vestiges of chains saws had left their mark.

The city had initiated a rigorous campaign of spraying DDT in the air from airplanes overhead to help defend the trees against the disease, but it didn't help. For a period of over ten years, more and more healthy trees became victims and began slowly shedding leaves and branches, with no hope of a recovery. The canopy of trees that once served to shade the town and add a certain charm and aesthetic beauty was transformed into pillars of death. Few yards escaped the barren look. Replanting was slow and seedlings were sorry substitutes for the once mighty tall lush live greenery. Not to mention the worry that any trees planted could end up dying as well all over again.

All those years of disseminating poison into the area was no match for the strength of Dutch Elm disease. I wondered what effects, if any, it had on the people living there. I wondered if we'll ever know.

In the summer of 1971, as I started my last year of undergraduate school, my father surprised me with a phone call. In four years he'd never called, let alone come all the way out to Utah to pay his son a visit. Mom wrote once in a blue moon, but not Dad.

"Stephen, we really need to talk. I have some bad news. I have been diagnosed with cancer and they tell me I only have about six more months to live. I've been to Kansas City, to KU Med Center. I've been to the best doctors in Tulsa. I get the same answer everywhere I go. Six months, that's all they give me."

"What?" I gasped. "What do you mean?" I was hoping somewhere in this conversation there was more which was better news. This was too sudden and too cruel.

He gave up smoking. He was no longer an alcoholic. His law business practice was prospering again. He'd started exercising, which he hadn't done for years. He and Mom were happy, or at least it seemed that way. He'd gotten his life back like he wanted it. Then this? Why?

"I have an inoperable brain tumor," he went on," and there is cancer in my lungs. It's just a matter of time. I will be taking chemotherapy, but they don't give me much chance."

"I should come home and be with you then. If your days are limited I want to spend them with you."

"No. That won't be necessary. You stay there in school. You come home for Christmas just like you always do. We'll talk then."

I continued to protest, but it fell on deaf ears. I loved him and I realized I wouldn't get to see him very many more times. Things were OK at school and I needed to focus on keeping it that way. Only then did it occur to me maybe going to college so far away from family was not a good idea. His news caught me totally unprepared. I would have never seen it coming.

I made a quick trip home anyway, and I took Angie with me to meet my family, Dad, my mother, my brother and my sister. They'd never met before. I wanted to see my Dad before Christmas. I thought,"What if he didn't make it that long?" We were there just a day, long enough to take a quick drive through town for Angie to see where I grew up and then we went to the hospital to visit Dad.

I barely recognized him. He was gaunt, grey, and visibly weak. He'd lost a lot of weight from all parts of his body. His face, his arms, his frame were all a fraction of what he used to look like. Worse than that there was no twinkle in his blue eyes when we walked in. He was semi-delirious. He was fading away, almost, but not quite already gone completely. I could tell that right away this wasn't the Dad I knew. It wasn't even the Dad I had talked to a few weeks ago. He was declining fast. The cancer and the drugs were taking its toll on him.

"Hi. Dad."

There was silence. Then finally… "Uh. Son. Stephen."

"Yeah. It's me, Dad." I wanted to talk with him. I wanted to say everything stored up inside me. I wanted to tell him how sorry I was I yelled at him when I was 14 and lost that golf tournament. I wanted to thank him for all the times he was there for me. I wanted to ask his forgiveness for all the embarrassment and grief I caused him. But, it was too late.

"Dad. This is Angie, my fiancée."

He nodded, barely.

"A-n-g-i-e....Angie" He spelled her name and said her name, but no more.

We stayed and talked a while, but it was clear he was slow and not aware of much. He understood a little and he would repeat words back to us but without adding anything to what I had said.

I kissed him and we left. I stopped just outside the room after his door was closed, leaned against it and bawled. He went from a seemingly healthy man to near death since the last time we were together in only a few months. He had recovered from his diabetes. He had stopped smoking and drinking alcohol. He had restored his faith in God. He had a new outlook on life. And now it was not nearly enough. The years I had hoped to spend with him in a renewed, closer and more mature father-son relationship had just gone up in smoke.

My father lay there dying in a Coffeyville Memorial Hospital, coincidentally the same hospital where I was born. I knew I would never see him alive again after that day. He had been everything to me. He had done more for me than anyone else. I owed him so much, and there was no way to thank him, or pay him back. I suddenly felt lost in a way I had never felt before. I had never lost a Dad before. I never would again. It wasn't fair.

I had battled back from losing a career with the Air Force. I had battled back from being put on academic probation at college. When something was taken away from me I figured out a way to move on and put it behind me. This was different. I couldn't replace my Dad. This was forever, and I knew it. I had lost my Aunt Mary, and, of my grandparents three had recently departed, but I wasn't as close to them. It was too late to make up the time to be close to Dad again, and that was what hurt the most. We stayed away from each other during the times we probably needed to be together the most.

One glowing ember that continued to burn in me was the confusion and the pressure when we returned back to Utah about what to do with my two girl friends. I had one in Kansas, Janis, whom I had known since 7th grade, and we had always kept in touch and dated whenever I was home for the holidays, or any break from school. Angie and I had been together for three years. I was engaged to Angie but the news of Dad's health and his imminent demise clouded everything.

I could marry Angie. I could marry Janis. I could let them both go and keep searching. I was anticipating the coming of a huge void in the wake of my father's death, and I felt it was urgent to be ready to fill that void when he passed away.

And then there was the impending question of what I was going to do to make a living. My career paths were simple but quite different. I could pursue golf as a profession. I knew more about it, and demonstrated more talent and skill than any other thing I knew.

Or, I could become a psychologist, an idea which fascinated me, and I thought I would be very good at it, but I would need a master's and probably a doctorate. Where would I get the money for that? Dad once mentioned setting up a college fund to me, but I knew he didn't. Whatever I did, it was going to be up to me.

These questions loomed larger and more significant as the fall semester moved toward its ending. I called Janis and asked her if she would be there at Dad's funeral as a favor to me. She acquiesced.

There was always something very calming about her. I was going to need that. She was good about things like that. If I ever needed her, I knew I could count on her. That's the way she was.

One night the pressure reached a boiling point, a level beyond anything I had ever known. I lay in bed tossing and turning, sweating profusely, as words kept repeating themselves in my head. Marry Janis….marry Angie…..be a psychologist….be a golf pro. The words were incessant, inescapable, and unanswerable. They rang loudly in my head over and over. God help me. What am I going to do? The room seemed to be heating up. The bed was moving but I wasn't. The room was as black as coal and getting darker. Time seemed to move too slowly. When was I going to go to sleep? I sensed that the walls were moving closer to me. The ceiling was dropping. My space was becoming more confined adding pressure to every emotion I felt. The air in the room was not enough to breathe regularly. My heart pounded and my chest heaved gasping for air, to no avail.

Somewhere around 4 am there came an odd stillness, as if the air in the room had been in a wind tunnel at a hundred miles an hour and all of a sudden the air currents stopped completely. The darkness grew lighter in my bedroom. My body, which had become exhausted from hours of the growing tension of every muscle getting tighter and tighter, suddenly relaxed. My breathing slowed, then stopped. My eyes were wide open.

Two decisions were now as lucid as anything I had ever known. They came smoothly, effortlessly and naturally into my consciousness after long hours of being lost in a merciless wrenching quandary. These two thoughts set a direction for the course of my life. I would become a golf professional. I would marry Janis. I accepted these two decisions as absolute certainty.

I never looked backed questioning where they came from. I began moving forward from that night. I was OK with my choices. I sure didn't want to go through that night's torment ever again.

Beginning that fall semester I decided I needed something to channel my thoughts into, my creative energies. I rented a used upright piano for $30 a month for two months, and played it every chance I had.

I was enchanted by the song "Stairway to Heaven" by Led Zeplin, and had been playing it my mind for days. I taught myself to play it on the piano. It was a good mental escape, but it didn't help with my most pressing problems.

When the house was empty I would play for hours, but there were no solutions hiding under the keyboard.

Breaking my engagement with Angie would be hard, but I was compelled to follow through with my "Big Decisions." I needed to find the right time to tell her.

I was nearly at the corridor of the next stage of my life. I had to go forward. I had to have a plan. Graduation was only months away. It was time for decisions to be made. I would marry Janis, not Angie. I knew I was taking a risk because I hadn't asked Janis yet. But, I had an inner confidence about the outcome of that.

22

IN NOVEMBER, I got a call from Mom that Dad had died. I flew home by myself. GrandDaddy Weiss was there at our house when I arrived. Janis did attend the funeral as I had previously asked of her. We spent some time together after the ceremony, but I mostly had to spend time with my family for the rest of that day.

The next day I took her to Big Hill. We sat on a small merry-go-round, and I pushed us around a few times. Then I held her hand.

"Janis, will you to marry me? I love you and I want to spend my life with you."

She accepted willingly.

I immediately made the obvious realization I was simultaneously engaged to two very fine, very wonderful and very different young women. I had made my mind up previously to select Janis. I had to let Angie know that piece of bad news. I couldn't wait. I was around family and friends after Dad's funeral the rest of the day and couldn't get to a phone or a quiet space with so much going on.

I went back to Kansas City with Janis, and planned to fly out of there to return back to Utah. Soon after we walked into Janis's apartment I picked up the phone.

"Angie, Steve. Bad news. This is going to be really hard. I hate to have to say this. I'm breaking our engagement."

"Why? What happened?" I could hear here voice lose its firmness and start to crackle.

"I asked Janis to marry me. I've decided to go with her. That means I have to give up being with you."

"When are you coming home? Here, you know?"

"Tonight."

"Let's talk when you get back. I think you are tired. You're emotional about your Dad. Let's talk about all this when you get back here. OK?"

"I've made up my mind, Angie. I want you to know that, but, yes, OK, we'll talk, face to face. Tonight. As soon as I get back there."

Pause……. "Steve. I love you."

"I know. I love you, too." Janis was looking at me during this conversation. This was not an easy thing.

"Then why are you doing this to me?"

"That's what we need to talk about. It's hard to do this over the phone. Let's just do all the talking face to face when I get back there. OK?"

I eventually got her to hang up. She was crying, and I was feeling badly. I thought to myself *this was not going to be easy to do.*

The dualities of life - of pain and joy, sorrow and happiness, life and death, hope of a future life and it's being ended prematurely – I saw them all that weekend. They all ran through my mind and my heart, one at a time then blurred together. I lost my father. I chose a life partner. Was it too much too fast? I knew there were no answers.

Back in Logan, having just kissed Janis goodbye hours earlier, late that night I went to Angie's apartment. She was up, franticly pacing, chain smoking, awaiting my arrival.

"What are you doing to me? To us?" She was teary eyed.

Puffy red eyes from hours of tears. "What do I have to do now to make it up to you? What did I do wrong? You can't just do this to me. Didn't I mean anything to you?"

"Angie. Settle down. Let's sit down." She was hanging on my shoulders not wanting to pull away.

"I had to make a choice. I love both of you, but that won't work for either one of you and it's not fair. You had done nothing wrong. There is nothing you can do or say. There is nothing wrong with you. It's me. I'm screwed up.

It's not your fault. You are the innocent victim here. I have to say goodbye to one of you. I have to. You see that don't you?"

"But, why her and not me? That's what I don't understand."

"I don't understand it either. I can't explain it to you. I have to just do it, break it off. I can't be with both of you. I can't marry both of you. I can't be with both of you in two places at one time. I can't be loyal to two of you. I can't, I can't, I can't. It's not fair to either one of you."

"Why don't you get some sleep and we'll talk it through tomorrow. You're very upset, very emotional. Hell. You lost your father, what do expect? You're not yourself. Now's the wrong time for this. Don't you agree? Can't you see that?"

At that point she had become calmer than I was. I realized at that moment I had never severed a relationship with anyone. I was always the one who had been dumped. I'd never done this before.

I was always on the other side. I knew how she felt. I knew exactly how she felt. And, it's crummy. Helpless. Powerless. Crazy.

I felt rotten. My stomach curled up like I had been swallowing rocks. It was my fault. I had been eating my cake and having it, too. Two girls, two parts of the country, it was explainable. College and home were a long ways apart. It wasn't planned. It wasn't devious. All along it seemed harmless and justifiable. I did this to myself and I didn't have to pay for it, Angie suffered the consequences. How gutless was that?

I looked at her and drew a big breath. "Angie. No matter how hard you try. No matter what you say. No matter how wrong I am. It's my fault, blame me entirely. But, what I say stands. I will be with her, and I'm breaking up with you, and I'm sorry, so very sorry. It's been good – you and I. Best ever. Now I must say goodbye." I walked out shaking.

This was going to take time. These were permanent decisions, affecting all of us.

Coincidentally, the Rolling Stones came out with one of the most beautiful songs I'd ever heard, especially from them. The title was "Angie." Lyrics included the phrase "You Can't Say We Never Tried." That was fitting.

It was a quick engagement. Usually, folks would frown at getting tied so soon, but it wasn't really that soon at all. We'd known each other since we were thirteen. I'd eaten meals at her house dozens of times. I was well accepted by her family. It was going to be OK. We'd been dating every summer for years. We both went into the relationship with high hopes, lots of energy and tons of love and respect. I was marrying my best friend. But, I truly deeply loved her, too.

My room mate, Dick, was my best man and the rest of the groomsmen were local friends from high school. I was so nervous I had two fender benders in the two weeks prior to the big event.

Janis and I were married on a snowy Saturday, February 12. A song I wrote was played during the ceremony. We hired a piano player. I had to teach him how to play it, since I couldn't write music in sheet music form.

We had a beautiful wedding but there was no time for a honeymoon. That would have to wait until summer. I had to get back to college. We lived together in Utah a few months until I graduated. I was motivated to get out of there and took 27 hours to graduate on time. Mom brought Stuart and Sally to my graduation. That was the first time any of my family had come to Utah to visit me in four years. It was nice they came.

Janis came with me to class a few times, and watched me on the days I played golf, but she was used to working as a teacher in Kansas City, and got pretty bored pretty quickly. There were no teaching jobs available in Logan so she worked at a flower shop, planting little flowers into tiny pots for minimum wage. She was as glad as I was to get out of there.

I had a college golf tournament in Las Vegas against the University of Nevada and the University of Arizona. Janis came along despite protests from the coach that if we slept together I might not be at full strength. I didn't notice any difference and I played fairly well.

I had been to Vegas seven previous times for other golf events and always managed to find a little time to go to Caesar's Palace and play blackjack. And all seven times I won money, not big money, but I didn't bet big money because I didn't have big money. I played $2 bets, once in a while $5. When I was up $20 - $30 I got up and walked away.   I explained all this Janis with great pride that I was an excellent and wise, cautious and conservative gambler.

"No problem. I'll play a few hands and when I'm ahead we'll go have a drink and then take off. Promise. I always quit a winner."

"OK. But, you better be careful." She stood right behind me.

Janis knew nothing about blackjack or any other kind of gambling. Money was not something to be wasted on chance in the Herman house. My Dad gambled so I had a different philosophy. I put aside $150 in my wallet.

I reassured her again, "This is my gambling money. When it goes, we walk, although that's never happened. I'll even set a limit. Let's say, when I get to $150 ahead, we'll take off OK?"

She nodded, warily.

First hand I had a 10 and a 9, but the dealer had a pair of jacks. Bye bye to my first $2 chip. My second hand was a 5 and a 6. I doubled down and drew an ace. Dealer had 17 and I lost again.

"Ok, should be my turn now. I'll double my bet and get back even." I bet $4. But, I lost again. And again. And again. I lost 46 out of 50 hands and my $150 was gone.

"Do you have any idea how much I hate planting pots?" "The $150 I just sweated two weeks to make you just frittered away in thirty minutes. That's it. No more gambling for you. No more. You're never doing that again buster. Never! What a waste!" She was as adamant as I had ever seen her. I guess I would have seen it that way if I had been her.

Not only was my luck abysmal that night, but my timing couldn't have been worse. How could I lose so badly in front of Janis? Or, maybe I saved us a lot of money in the future not gambling it on anything else, but we clearly established a gambling policy early in our relationship. Zero tolerance. We never had that discussion again. Not until years later when I lost a bundle in the stock market.

23

I BEGAN MY golf professional career in San Antonio, Texas. It seemed like a good choice for both of us. Janis had an uncle who was able to help her get a teaching position. It was a good climate for golf. I was hired in a rather unusual way.

I looked up the PGA headquarters there, and contacted a man named George Albach, Executive Director. He told me the only job I might be interested in was over on the southeast side of town. My first job was at a municipal golf course, and I worked for the City of San Antonio. The interview was weird.

"Yes. I'm applying for the assistant golf position. Right. I played in college on a golf scholarship. I've been playing since I was 6 years old. I was a state champion in a junior tournament. Yes. I graduated just a few weeks ago from college at Utah State University. That's way out west from here. And a little north, too." I pointed toward what I thought was north. I was turned around pointing south, but no one said anything. I realized it later when I walked out and saw the sun.

The interview went very quickly, and I was told in a whisper I had the job, but I had to go through standard procedures. I sat there with an older black man, and a young Hispanic male, neither of which had any golf experience whatsoever, but they both went through the same interview that I went through. Then there was a lot of paper shuffling and finally I heard, "OK, Mr. Knapp. The assistant's job is yours. Next group please."

I was not at all familiar with equal opportunity laws. It certainly seemed like they stacked the deck in my favor, but that was just fine with me.

My first golf pro job only lasted a few weeks because my boss, Boyd Humphries, and I had serious philosophical differences, mostly about inventory procedures. I'm sure we had more than that to set us apart, but that was plenty enough.

Boyd told me, "What you are going to do is count everything in the shop when you start your shift. That's the first thing you do. He pointed his finger at me, at the clubs, the balls, the tees, the putters, the shirts, and then he pointed his finger at me again. "Then at the end of the day, you count the shop again. This sparked another round of finger pointing item by item and ending with me again. "What's missing is what is sold and it should equal the money you have in the cash register. Got it?"

"Yeah, I got it."

But, it turned out to be a huge waste of time to do things that way.

In my first eight hours on a very rainy day I sold 6 balls, 2 bags of tees, 1 glove and 2 candy bars.

I didn't need to spend a full hour counting things that no body even touched. It was simple. The receipts were there to tell about each purchase. Add them up and we're done. Let's go home.

"No. No. That's not how we do it. Mr. George Albach told me there was only one way to do this, and that's how we're going to do it."

"The only way for sure you know you didn't forget to write something down, or collect some money, is count everything."

"Beg your pardon, Mr. Humphries, with all due respect, sir, I don't forget things. I have a college degree. I smiled proudly."

"Well, I don't. But, that don't matter. Not one smidgen. Take this sheet here on this clip board and count everything in the shop. See what it adds up to when you extend all the prices. Fill it out and then we count the money and see if you have it right. They should be equal. If it don't, you did something wrong."

He had an old time adding machine where you press the numbers down and then crank the machine. It printed out a total. Everything in the store was added together one category at a time.

His wife, Marge, had come by just to talk. She sat there smoking a cigarette and smiled dreamily at him while we went through all of this. She liked to talk about her three cats. They had no children. He drank over 20 cup of coffee a day. I could see we were going to have a lot of discussions and I probably wasn't going to win many of them.

I took too many short cuts and made a too many mistakes. I finished quickly, maybe too quickly.

"OK. Let's see. Look at this, now." I was finished and ready to call it a day.

He read it over carefully. "Seems like they didn't teach you how to count so good up there at college, young feller. You're a dollar and twenty two cents short."

"Here," I reached into my pocket. I gave him five quarters and said "Keep it. Put it in the deposit. Keep the pennies."

"NO. NO. NO." He screamed at me. "That's not how you do it. Go back and count everything in the shop again and let's see where you made a mistake."

"You want me to spend another 45 minutes counting to see if I can find another dollar and twenty two cents? Are you kidding?"

"That's exactly what I want you to do. That's the only way we are going to solve this."

I considered myself a fairly easy going, fairly easy to get along with sort of guy. But, I recognized this was just not going to work for me.

After two weeks we mutually decided it was best if I moved on. I couldn't work there, not in a blue moon. I had an innate sense of efficiency. I hated waste. I hated doing things that didn't make sense, especially when there was a better way. I could think of ten better ways for everything I did all day long. This place was a classic throwback to the Middle Ages, maybe Neanderthal ages, but it just wasn't for me.

On a Saturday with little important to do, Janis and I decided to discover downtown San Antonio, and the Alamo, and the Riverwalk, and the famous space needle. We made a day of it.

"Saturday, in the park, I think it was the 4th of July,…" a classic Chicago song was playing on the radio. Walking down the street close to the Alamo I saw a design on the pavement that struck a chord in my memory.

I stopped dead in my tracks. "Janis, look at that. See that "A" in the sidewalk. If I'm right….well…let's just see… If we go through that door, turn right, go just past the huge fire place and look down, you'll see a baby alligator crawling around in a pit."

"Are you serious? Are you psychic, or just joking?"

"Come on. Follow me." I took her hand.

The image on the side walk was as clear in my mind as the day on our way to Mexico when my family stayed in San Antonio when I was 10. To certify my memory wasn't tilted, we looked down in the lower rock pit together and sure enough, the baby alligator was there. Not the same one I saw before when I was there the last time, but one just like it. Nothing had changed. Hotel Ancira was just as I remembered it.

"Wow." Janis was impressed. Photographic memory was working quite well that day.

I dressed up in character and worked as Mr. Scrooge for the Christmas holidays at a department store close to our apartment, and in January I got a real assistant pro's job at Abilene Country Club, in Abilene, Texas.

Janis had a good teaching position in San Antonio at Alamo Heights which she had to give up to make the move with me. There were no teaching positions available in Abilene dues to the abundance of colleges there. She worked at a bank for a short time and then some private schools, but nothing permanent. Later she found a job with a home for wayward girl's and became their Executive Director.

I had inherited Dad's Chevrolet Impala. He had put studs on the tires as a precaution for slick icy Kansas streets. They came in handy in Utah, but I wanted to take them off when we were in San Antonio. The chances of ice were zero, and they went "clackety – clackety- clack" everywhere I drove. Janis said wait until they wear completely down.

On a very rainy dark sultry night I was glad I had them on. I was on the freeway when a car came to my left side and hit my car.

Bam, and again, Bam. And once more, Bam ! The third time I lost control of the car and was heading toward a barrier with another freeway underneath it. I hit the brakes as hard as I could and stopped inches from going through the barrier. The driver hit me in the rear panel, the side door and the front panel before driving on and disappearing. Several cars stopped to see if I was OK. They were witnesses and told the police how the guy tried to pass me when there was no lane empty. He also sideswiped the car beside me. Those old tire studs probably saved my life that night.

I had a job I really liked in Abilene, but it only paid $4 an hour and I work 70 hours a week. We scraped by for almost a year and then Janis was pregnant. She knew it within weeks. She wanted to have her first child naturally, with me in the delivery room, and Abilene hospital ideology had not yet accepted the concept of "natural childbirth," so I had to find another job in a more progressive community.

I got lucky and we were soon on our way to Bartlesville, Oklahoma, and I would work at Hillcrest Country Club for the next six years. It was good because we lived only 45 minutes from Coffeyville, so Janis and I could see our families every so often.

We moved our stuff to Oklahoma in a U-haul truck, with Janis's gold Camero towed behind it. Janis drove in my old Impala, I drove the truck. After we found an apartment and got everything moved, we had to return the truck and the trailer hitch back to the dealer.

I disconnected the trailer hitch and put it into the back of the truck. I lifted the hitch, stood it up on the truckbed and immediately passed out. Janis saw me on the ground and moved to quickly steady the hitch before it fell on top of me.

"Help. Help! Somebody help me. NOW! HELP!" She screamed with all her might. Janis was not nearly strong enough to hold the several hundred pound frame, but she somehow kept it balanced just long enough. She was pregnant, too. Some guys ran to help her and it was all over before I came to.

"Wha, wha, what am I doing here?" I was on the ground looking up at Janis.

"You're a lucky man, Steve. You passed out on me. I can't believe that. Thanks you guys, I guess he's all right now."

"Sure. See ya'."

I was watching two men walk away and didn't have a clue what had just happened.

I guess I didn't get enough oxygen when I was lifting it. I was fortunate it didn't crush me. To this day Janis tells me "breathe" when I lift anything heavy.

24

OUR FIRST DAUGHTER, Marysa, was born a few months later without complications, and two years following we had a son, Weslee. Both were born with Janis and I working together in the delivery room. The Lamaze classes were a big help. Our family was growing in size rapidly, having doubled in two years time.

Janis had mentioned several times she wanted four children. I guess since she was the first of five in her family that four was a number she would be comfortable with. Two seemed to me like the right number for us and so we stayed with the idea of raising just two.

Funds were short and Janis was worried she would have to find a full-time baby sitter and go back to teaching right after his birth. Fortune favored me and I won a local small golf tournament. The $1400 I won bought her another six months of getting to stay at home. I worked long hours, and we didn't have much but we were blissfully happy.

After over four years there it seemed to me that I should be ready to move up, but my boss wasn't leaving so I had to find a club that would hire me as their head pro. This was not a simple task to accomplish. I had to convince some board of directors could handle all the responsibilities in their club. And there had to be an opening, which in the mid-west was not very often. Most importantly, I had to win over all the competition when there was an opening, and there were hundreds to compete against for one job.

The first thing I had to do was get an interview. Only a handful of applicants were chosen, usually by a country club board of directors who were elected from their membership. After all the interviews were completed then one head pro would be selected.

In the next two years I had a grand total of three interviews for head pro jobs at country clubs, which wasn't bad considering the sparse number of opportunities. I interviewed in Topeka, Kansas. I had an interview in Midland, Texas. I had an interview in Ardmore, Oklahoma. When you only get one shot every six months, and that interview lasts about two hours each time, there is a lot of pressure. For exact reasons I'll never know, I was not chosen for any of them. My guess is I looked too young, and had no head pro experience, or maybe I was too stiff. Not surprisingly, all the men who won the head pro positions that I didn't get went on to have very successful careers. I came so close.

I gave over 2000 golf lessons and played some very good rounds of golf. But, I was still very stiff at times. I looked very tense and not relaxed. I walked and carried myself awkwardly. My mouth was open and my jaw stuck out often. I knew this because I saw pictures and home movies where I barely recognized myself. On film I looked completely differently that the way I imagined myself. I'd seen my mouth open, jaw jutting out, jerky off balance walk. Maybe Mrs. Ketchum, my ballroom dance instructor was right. I WAS stiff.

But why?

I made my boss upset at me a number of times when I did not do what he wanted me to do. I was torn between pleasing my boss and my members when they seemed to be at odds with each other and I was in between.

My memory was superb and I could easily recall the names of over seven hundred members and their families. The little details I had down pat.

I could find any one of over 250 member's golf bags stored in the back room of the shop without having to look up their location. I knew the rules of golf backwards and forwards. I knew the fundamentals of the golf swing and could give individual lessons, as opposed to the one-size-fits-all variety, which were precisely helpful only for the person I was teaching at that time. For some reason it was the common sense issues and good judgment that seemed to always betray me.

Cecil Magana, a very wealthy club member who had a short fuse occasionally was with some of his guests and I went out on the course to speed them up. A round of golf at Hillcrest Country Club should be completed in four hours or less.

"Hey. Excuse me. I need you to play faster. They're waiting behind you."

I wasn't very tactful. I just blurted it out.

My boss and Cecil nearly got into a fight over it. A few days later I yelled at Mr. Magana's son, Travis, who worked for us for a while. He forgot to turn on the battery chargers to the golf carts. This meant the carts would run out of power and strand the players all over the course with no transportation to get back to the club house.

I plugged them in myself to get it done right. But, I over reacted. I didn't need to yell at him. He just needed to be trained better, and that was my job.

My photographic memory had another related talent - I had a similar knack for remembering sounds and voices.

"Ring, ring. Good morning. Steve speaking. Hillcrest Golf Shop, how may I help you?"

"Put me down for….."

"Oh, Hi. Dr. Emmott. Regular group, usual tee time at 10:32 am this Saturday?"

"Yep, thanks."

"I got you down. Thank's for calling, Dr. See you then." Hillcrest Golf Shop……."

I would write down on the tee time sheet – Emmott, Winslow, Hardin, McPhail, and quickly answer the next call.

Dr. Emmott was a urologist, Bill Winslow sold insurance, Dr Hardin was a dentist specializing in braces and Bill McPhail was into construction and oil well drilling.

I knew everyone's name after I had heard their voice utter the first syllable. I knew their likes and dislikes. Who they played with. Who they sat beside on the golf cart.

What the names of all their families were. What colors they wore in their choice of slacks and shirts. What their handicap was. I knew their swing. Their interests. Their habits. I knew my customers well. They were a giant family to me – about 1500 people altogether. I spent more time with them than I did at home with my wife and kids. That's just how it was. An assistant golf pro makes many sacrifices.

The frustrations of being the number two pro and not able to move up continued to stick in my craw. One day I got so upset I quit Hillcrest Country Club to work at a Godfather's pizza place, but a few hours later I asked for my old job back and got it. I was perplexed and disappointed. I was trapped in a career place wanting to advance to the next level and no one would let me. I had to be patient, which I usually was, but there seemed to never be an end to my waiting.

I felt Janis and I were treading water, watching our friends move up in the world in status and financial gain. We both had college degrees and our present financial status qualified us for food stamps, but we were far too proud to consider that option.

It was no longer good enough to be content with staying home, watching "Dallas," on TV and never going out to enjoy a night on the town. Rarely did we eat out or see a movie or go on a nice vacation. We couldn't afford those things.

I took an offer at a club in Idabel, Oklahoma. The members there called it Idabel, America. It was a very small town in southeast Oklahoma. I was not just the golf pro, I was club manager, activity planner, swimming pool director, and all the food and beverage headaches were mine, which took up most of my time. I moved there by myself and saw my family on certain weekends until I could see my way through on this new position. The people there were great, and very friendly, but in the short span of six months, the clubhouse was broken into and robbed three times, costing me thousands of dollars. The trailer house I was living in next to the club house was also broken into and ransacked.

There were racial riots in the town. A school was torched. A radio station was burned to the ground. To me, this was not a safe place to bring my family to settle down in.

Of course, the members accepted all the activities as unfortunate, but not a big deal. I saw it as potentially dangerous for raising a family. At the first chance I had, I took another similar job as a club manager, which happened to be in my old home town in Coffeyville, Kansas.

My new contract read in part…."you will be responsible for the worker's compensation for all the employees." I read it. I knew what it meant. I had just the right guy in mind to help me get a policy. I needed to spread my business around. It was a small town. Carl Garrison, local insurance agent and club member, would get me a worker's comp policy and make a few bucks.

But, good ol' Carl was out of town. "When will he back?" I asked the lady answering the phone in his office. I needed to talk to him.

"It will be next Wednesday. That's in five days. OK?"

"OK." I could wait a few days.

I felt it was important to give him the business. I wanted to speak to him, Carl, so he knew it was me giving him the business.

The next day Toni came up to me. She was a waitress at the club, one of my 25 employees. She told me she hurt her back lifting a tray of food serving it to the Read family last night. I told her to go to her doctor and have it checked if it was started really bothering her.

Toni was the oldest person on the staff. I didn't hire her, I inherited her all along with the crew. I was too new to get things squared away to deal with personnel issues right off the bat. I had inventory and Wednesday night buffet to plan for, and I had golf lessons to give.

Toni was small, short, bent over, crabby, and not well liked by the crew. She was in her late 50's, grey hair, spindly legs, wrinkly arms, and wore too heavy make-up.

Toni called me the next day. She couldn't come to work because she had too much back pain. Had to stay in bed all day she told me.

Next day Toni called. She had to go to the doctor. He put her in the hospital for tests. Strained back muscles, severe strain. Will be out at least a week. I was short a waitress for a week. Great.

Toni never came back to work. Too much pain. Went back into the hospital again.

I talked to Carl who finally got back in town. I told him about Tony.

"Sorry, Steve. Can't help you with that. I can work up the policy. I can't date it back before her accident. You've got to take care of her on your own."

What have I got myself into now? I was thinking I could be ruined.

I went see my uncle Frank. He'd bailed Dad out of jail. Now I needed him to bail me out of this problem. He said,"Wait. Do nothing. Say nothing. Just wait."

The writing was on the wall that I was never going to be a head golf pro at a big, prestigious country club, which is what I had been working for seven years. I got the notion it was time to change careers. Get a real job with benefits. Spend time with the kids who I never saw much awake. I was working from 6 am to 1 or 2 am, seven days a week. No vacation. No days off. No retirement. No insurance. It wasn't very lucrative or otherwise rewarding. That was not for me any more. And I didn't want to deal with Toni.

My thoughts were to get a job with Phillips 66. I had met seventeen vice-presidents while I was in Bartlesville, because that was their headquarters. My idea was to work for Phillips and go back to college and get an MBA while I was working. The MBA was crucial. No oil company would want a golf pro with a psychology degree. It took a few months of knocking on doors, but I finally landed a position with them.

There were only a couple of problems.

"Steve. I love you and I'll move anywhere in the country with you except two places – New York or Houston." Janis had told me her wishes many times. New York was too congested and Houston was too dangerous, too much crime, according to her. It didn't matter what her reasons were. She wasn't going to go there. So guess where Phillips said they'd send me?

My job offer with Phillips 66 was in Houston, Texas. Janis and I argued but in the end I took it. It was my chance for change. A new direction. A new future. Better than I was facing if I stayed doing what I was doing. It meant in increase in pay, and they would pay for 90% of my education. But, it was a 1000 mile commute. I had to do it. It was my best option. If I was going to work for a big oil company I would need more education. A double major undergraduate degree in psychology and sociology was not going to cut the mustard.

She stayed in Coffeyville, and her Mom and Dad helped raise our kids. She also began getting her masters degree in education. I enrolled at the University of Houston, and began working shift work at the Houston Chemical Complex where I wore a hard hat and ear plugs and made extruded polypropylene plastic.

Once a month I flew home for four days and enjoyed being with my family. I became a regular passenger on Southwest Airlines. When the University of Houston began its next session I took sixteen hours of graduate school per semester for the next two years straight. I graduated with a 3.5 GPA and I had my MBA.

I'd been working a job with shift work on a rotating monthly schedule so I worked 6 days, 7 evenings and 7 graveyard shifts with a few days off in between. I averaged 4 hours of sleep per night for over two years and I had to miss 25% of my classes because I was working during scheduled class time. But, classmates and professors all worked with me to help me get through it.

At Phillips I worked with a completely different kind of people than ever before. I was used to doctors, and lawyers, and corporate executives, and retired old men, and women married to men wealthy enough they could play golf and not worry about finances.

In Houston I was surrounded by laborers with high school diplomas. They were suspicious of me, and jealous, in the beginning. Some thought I was a spy. It was a culture shock for me. I clearly didn't fit in, and I was a "short-timer." When I got my MBA I would be gone. They were "lifers." This was as good as it would ever be for them.

And it wasn't that bad. $11.20 an hour plus 8 hours overtime each week and some weeks more overtime than that. Benefits were the best I had ever had. That was for sure. I had to wait a year before I could invest in the 401-k, but I took advantage of it as soon as I qualified. I had medical benefits, two weeks paid vacation. It was not great, and it was a trade-off. I was away from my family most of the time. I hoped it was a short term loss for a long term gain. I was totally committed to it. I would do whatever it took.

At the end of a shift cycle of six mornings, seven evenings, and seven graveyards with a few days off in between I'd leave the plant at 7 am and driving to Houston Hobby Airport. In an airport restroom I would shave, clean my hands and face, change out of my work clothes and into a pair of slacks and a golf shirt and board a Southwest Airlines flight to Tulsa, OK. A shuttle bus took me to Bartlesville, and Janis would pick me up there mid afternoon. I would stay four days and fly back for another 28 days work cycle before returning again.

The plant was a union shop, Oil Chemical and Atomic Workers (OCAW) and most of the workers belonged. I did not sign up, which didn't make me very popular when I was asked about it. They paid their dues, which I did not pay, and I got the same benefits that they got.

I learned Texas was a right to work state, and I was not forced to join. In time I became friends with most of the crew I worked with. I adopted their language. For example, if they told me to check an air line, it could be "blocked off" or "blocked up" or "blocked out" or just "blocked." It all meant the same thing. I just had to close a valve.

It was hot, noisy and tiresome work. The plastic I worked with was over 500 degrees just before it was cooled and made into tiny pellets. But, it was honorable employment and the guys and the women I worked with were all good people.

One night around midnight I was at the plant. I was working 11 – 7, the graveyard shift. Most of every hour I sat watching controls, extruders, and various equipment designed to make polypropylene pellets. I was assigned to Train 1 that night.

It would run for the entire shift without a change, or need a shutdown as long as I keep it in line.

That's what I did as an operator. I got it going, and kept it going within the set points. If I screwed up, the quality or quantity was off spec. I couldn't allow that. I was trained to keep it in line all the time.

Most nights it was a simple matter of checking every so often and then sat down and try to stay awake. It was deafening because of the extruders and the reactors. I wore ear plugs which hardly shut out all the noise, but they helped.

That night I was in my own world, thinking about a beat in my mind, a drum beat. Ta, da, da, dum, da, da, da, dum, da, da, da. I kept it steady and realized I could put words to it. I started writing down words that went with the beat. I used a pad for notes about the plastic I was making.

In an hour I had it. I was thinking it would be cool to have a group of guys say the words with the drum beat in the background. It would sound different. Like a song with no music. A song with words but no instruments, except for the drum. I liked the idea and thought about it until it was time to go. No. It was too different, I decided. Too radical. No one would ever like that. No one would want to record something like that. Or listen to something like that. I had been in radio for four years and listened to a lot of radio after I left KGGF. Nothing I ever heard was like the idea I just had. It didn't even have a name. You couldn't call it music. I ripped off the paper, put the words in my pocket and walked out to my car. Shift was over.

I never did anything about my idea. It would be many years before "rap" was popular. I don't even think the word had been invented yet. I was ahead of my time. But, nobody knew it.

I began working in the fall of 1981. Soon after I started there Phillips put a freeze on hiring. The country and the city were feeling economic hard times. 15,000 engineers in Houston were out of work. The oil industry was going through tough major adjustments. The economy continued to worsen.

Six months after I had been working for Phillips I still had no seniority, I was still last on the list of new hires. I had to worry about being laid off which added another layer of pressure to everything going on with classes and traveling to see Janis and the kids.

On my usual monthly trip home to Coffeyville for four days, I met with Frank in his office about Toni.

He talked the Club into paying for her medical bills. It was finally over for me. I didn't have that hanging over my head any longer. I had been lucky. I was OK, again. At least about that issue.

After I graduated with my MBA from the University of Houston, Clear Lake City campus, I was promoted out of the plant and into a cost accounting position for a few months and then I was accepted to be in a new class of trainees in the marketing department.

One of my last classes I had been doing research for a finance class paper. The professor wanted me to check out Eastern Airlines using Value Line which was loaded with financial information. I found it in the library. It was a book with 1700 companies and it listed every financial number and graph I'd ever want to know and more. It contained stock prices over time, PE (price Earnings ratio), beta, profits, sales, number of employees, and on and on. I could see Eastern had been losing money for years. How could they do that and continue to operate?

That's what I had to answer. That was the point of the paper.

I thumbed through the pages glancing at their competition, TWA, United, Delta. Southwest seemed to be the most profitable. I flew them and they were always full, so no surprise there. Then I flipped randomly looking at charts.

I become focused on just charts. Flat. No good. Down from left to right, worse. Upwards left to right, good,

Good direction. Good sales, increasing stock price.

"I found a company that seemed to be growing vertically. No other company had a chart like it. Must be too good to be something that would continue.

I was thinking about some money I saved. $10,000. I could buy stock in this company and watch it grow.

Or, I could buy a car. I needed a car because my Dad's Impala is looking pretty bad and it has 160,000 miles on it.

I decided to shop for a car. I liked Thunderbirds. I found a deal in the papers for a used T-bird.

That stock couldn't keep going up like that. Just too precipitous. Too risky. Home Depot. Hmmmmmm. Never heard of it.

25

"YOU WHAT?" I called Janis to tell her I bought a nice used red Ford Thunderbird, two years old, for $8700.

"You don't buy a car without discussing it with me. What were you thinking of? How could you do that? I think you should take it back now. We've always discussed these kinds of things together first. What is the matter with you?"

It was true. We'd always discussed financial things together. This was a first. But, I was in Houston and my car was getting pretty shabby. I didn't take it back. Janis was furious with me. (Worse than that, if I'd spent $10,000 in Home Depot common stock, it would be worth over a million dollars today.) I kept the T-bird less than a year and lost a lot of money in the trade.

Finally, things changed for me for the better. I was transferred to Florida to run gas stations. It was winter, 1984, and life was looking up. I had a secure future. I could face new challenges with confidence. My family was going to be with me and we were all going to live happily ever after. I felt like maybe the All American Boy dream was just around the corner after all.

Janis and I went shopping for a nice business car. She did not like my Thunderbird at all. Maybe it was just that I bought it by myself. I think it was the concept, not the car. I got a nice new Chrysler. Now that I was on a mileage allowance I could afford a new car.

Janis also had a new car. It was small, a Chrysler Champ but it got great mileage. We drove to Leland for a family summer trip. Weather was great, food was great, and everyone had a good time. Janis bought a bumper sticker, I Love Leland, and put it on her car.

That fall Janis answered a knock at her door in Coffeyville. I had moved into an apartment in Fort Lauderdale, and she was planning to move to Florida with the kids when school was out.

Knock, knock.

"Hello. May I help you?" Janis did not recognize the young female at her door. But Coffeyville was full of friendly people and she didn't look threatening.

"Yeah. I want to know what you are doing with my boy friend?" She looked to be about 16 or 17.

"I don't know what you mean. Who is he" Janis was bewildered at this young girl's false accusation.

"You know, Leland. Leland Jones. He's my boyfriend.

What are you doing messin' around with him?"

"Why do you think I have anything to do with him? I've never heard of him. I've never seen him. What's your problem? I just don't understand?"

"It's your sticker on your car. It says you love Leland. What's that all about? Why do you have my boyfriend's name on your car?"

Janis couldn't hide her giggle. "I don't know your boyfriend. The sticker is about Leland, Michigan. We went there on vacation. We bought a bumper sticker in a gift shop that reminded us of the trip. That's all. Don't worry. It's just a coincidence."

"Oh. Whoops. I'm sorry." The girl turned around and left.

When Janis called me about her visitor we both had a good laugh. Some people in that small Kansas town never got out much. That was obvious.

26

IT WAS FAR from a good situation when I arrived in Ft Lauderdale. Lack of corporate interests and proper funding had relegated south Florida into a sorry heap of gas stations, most of which were so disgusting looking they had a different brand name – Waylo, which disguised their true ownership.

I decided to have a Christmas party for all the Phillips 66 employees and their spouses. It should have been a grandiose event. Most of the 120 people ignored the invitation and my reservations were way over the paltry 25 or so who made the effort to come. With all the no-shows, the evening did not have the warm feeling I had hoped to convey. Welcome to Florida and the real world, Steve-O!

I was way too naïve and trusting in the beginning. I just expected people to do what they were told. I was shocked that so many people stole money and food and credit cards. I made an A in my graduate managerial auditing class, but I never realized people would really use false credit cards, or forge checks, or just plain lie to my face. Dishonesty ran rampant in my local organization.

Graduate school did not give me the real world taste like being in south Florida and dealing with day to day problems. But, that was my job. I didn't do it very well and I had one boss that asked me if I would be better off doing something else. He could see I was intelligent, but I did not apply it in the most effective ways. I was working hard, but not working smart, and not getting the results I should have been getting.

I had put forth a great of effort and had not a lot to show for it. I promised him I'd do better, and I did.

I had fired a manager I caught stealing and in a show of loyalty to him the crew decided to quit and sabotage the store. It was the Pier 66 Plaza and Convenience store across the street from the Pier 66 Hotel in Fort Lauderdale. It was my biggest store. My pride and joy. It presented me with the opportunity to do what I had never done before. I managed it myself and slowly trained a new crew that stayed consistently with company policies, and adhered to my philosophies.

That gave me the confidence and experience I seriously needed to manage others. I had no fear of managers after that because they knew I could take over any time I had to. It gave me leverage and respect I had not enjoyed before then.

Mom came to Florida to visit us a few times. Once we went to Key West, with Aunt Hebby. Once she brought Sally and Stuart and we went to the Bahamas. Mom traveled well despite the news she had been diagnosed with cancer. She started chemotherapy when she got back to Kansas. She was very brave about it. 1986 she succumbed to the disease that had also taken her husband's life 15 years earlier. We flew to Leland to bid her farewell one last time.

It was such a unique and extraordinary occasion I wrote a poem about it:

One Winter's Day

She passed away one winter's day, it came as no surprise.
For time she bought with treatments
fought, four years to her demise.
Her valor earned, and, too, she learned just who her allies were.
The end defined, her course divined, the details now secure.

From near the start there came two
parts, two ceremonies planned.
The local friends who mourned her end
offered many helping hands.
The small town crowd for whom we're
proud all made the funeral blessed.
They came to share because they cared each wishing us their best.

But, here the story and its glory takes a twisting turn.
Beyond the grave, her soul was saved,
remains cremated to an urn.
Leland's grace, her chosen place, her family took her there.
Her childhood bond with memories fond
made a fitting, familiar air.

The sky was gray that shivering day, we gathered by the lake.
We huddled there and joined in prayers
the priest said for her sake.
We boarded a boat of choppy float just
family, the Father and the urn.
More prayers were made, and roses laid,
ashes sprinkled by each one in turn.

That moment God chose as we watched
the rose to open up the sky
The sun beamed through and we all knew
she came to say, "Goodbye."
The clouds then closed the deed disposed,
silence lead us back to shore.
Our mother dear now inside us here,
deep in our hearts forevermore.

I took my turn sitting on the cold boat's seats, sprinkling her ashes into Lake Michigan. I turned slightly and the wind blew my portion of the ashes into the faces and laps of many members of my family. We were more taken aback by the movement of the dark grey clouds overhead. They opened and made way for the light to shine down on us momentarily, and then closed and remained overcast the rest of the day.

The careless ashes spraying all about was left without comment until years later when Uncle Gary reminded us how un-seaworthy I had been that day.

27

I WON A trip for Janis and I to go to Portugal for a week. Later, I won a free week-end for the two of us at my choice of places. I ran up a hefty tab at an exclusive hotel called The Breakers in Palm Beach. Nice place. Things were going so well and I was getting good reviews, good raises. Things were looking up. And, then…

"Steve, I have some bad news." Dave Butler, my boss called me from Atlanta. Phillips management had decided it would be best to sell all their Florida assets. I had to make a decision soon. He couldn't tell me where we would move, or if I would be laid off. He was certain in a few months all my stations would be sold.

I asked him, "What's wrong? They're all making money. That's the object wasn't it?"

"Well, of course, but your margins are lower than in other parts of the country and your costs are relatively higher. Florida is a very expensive place to operate, you know that."

"OK." I understood. I felt very empty at that moment.

I thought to myself. Why is it every time things start to get better they don't stay that way very long?

I had to make a choice. If I stayed with Phillips, who knows where we'd end up? And maybe no where. The thought of moving my family was very disturbing to me and to them. It could be Oklahoma, or Texas, or maybe they didn't have a spot for me and I would have to start all over with another company.

I was sure in my mind they would transfer me to Bartlesville. No one told me, it was just a hunch. But, I was so certain I knew it was just a matter of time.

Corporations do not move in tandem with family activities. Marysa wanted to be in cheerleading. School would be starting soon. With my best intentions in mind I sent Marysa to Coffeyville to live with her grandparents and start the school year there. She could do her cheerleading and I was sure we would be moved to Bartlesville soon, and we would be rejoined at that point.

Marysa did spend a year with her grandparents living in Coffeyville. Then she moved back to Florida to be with us. I'd already given up on Phillips. They gave me no choice.

I thought I might need more education, so I began attending Florida Atlantic University and enrolled in a masters program in public administration, taking night classes.

I made a phone call. I quickly had an interview with Texaco and I was hired. I had to take a slight drop in salary, but, the only one that had to make any adjustments with this decision was me. Texaco was in growth mode. In retrospect, I should have contacted Shell, Mobil, Amoco, Exxon, and Chevron too see what they offered, but I took the first and only offer I sought and that was that. I didn't look further than not having to move the whole family.

I knew the area. I knew the Florida market. I had increased responsibilities and I thought it would work out great. Texaco was certainly well known and they had excellent benefits. I had a future again.

There was an opening for me because of a large corporate acquisition of more than 100 stores mostly located in Florida. Soon I was Operations Supervisor for 36, then 52, then 72 Texaco stores in south Florida. I was responsible for the profits and losses, expenses, maintenance, gas pricing, environmental issues and the performance of over 400 employees. I looked at 72 profit and loss statements monthly, and other reports which were updated weekly.

This was heaven for me. I liked the challenge of it. I managed it well. I had the respect and cooperation of those who worked under me. I made good decisions and profits climbed while expenses fell. I was rolling. I had a nice company car.

My boss was aiming his sights on retirement and didn't want to rock any boats. He was also ill from suffering from diabetes. He had his own agenda and shoved too much work on me. I was doing his job and mine. I worked too hard for too long. I was working unbelievable hours again, 100 hour a week with inescapable stress.

And I was in class three nights a week at Florida Atlantic University. It was too much.

One day my boss called into his office. "Knapp. Come in here. Sit and listen. Don't ask any questions. I'm reassigning you. I don't know what the hell you're doing. Arlene's taking your place. You go take care of the monitor wells and I don't want to see you around here at all. Get out!"

His secretary, Arlene, undermined me at strategic moments and I was unaware and too gullible to see what she had been doing. That one day my boss was furious and took away all my power.

Only my environmental duties remained with me and he shifted everything else to her. All the projects I had on going went to a halt. The four maintenance technicians reporting me were now on their own. The ten supervisors who ran 6 – 10 stores each were off limits. I wasn't allowed to talk to them.

Her prior qualifications included being a former hair stylist with no college education. I was crushed that he could consider her, but I did not know what she had been telling him. Even so, he was a fool for not giving me more loyalty, as I had given him.

This came as a total shock to me. The timing couldn't have been worse. We had just built a new house and Janis was pregnant.

Strangely, it must have been obvious. Janis figured it out. She saw it coming and warned me to be wary of Arlene. I didn't listen. My job change upset Janis so badly she had a miscarriage driving to work two days later. For several months all I did was examine monitor wells and record the environmental data at all our stations. The raise I had been given before everything went crazy was rescinded. My company car, a new Ford Taurus station wagon, had been taken away. I got another car but it was a sedan with 50,000 miles on it. Everything that was happening made no sense. My world was ripped apart. Something had to give. Once again, when things seems to be going well, a disaster hits me blindside. It happens over and over throughout my life. Why?

Later, the truth came out. I was reassigned, again, and the secretary, Arlene, was fired along with two others in the office. My boss requested to take me with him to his new job, and he continued to be my boss in a different office, working in a different class of trade. It was very confusing to not know if he was on my side or against me.

Things began to look up. My raise was restored and my workload had been reduced from the craziness I had before the bottom fell. I got a new company car. I was back in good graces, but not completely. There was personnel file damage that would never escape me, even though I did not deserve it.

On July 26, 1990, our government passed the American Disability Act. Title III of this new law cost Texaco a huge amount of money. The public had to be accommodated for access to our facilities. The new law had a direct impact of my job responsibilities and kept me busy assisting in all the necessary changes.

For example, ramps had to be constructed so wheel chair customers could reach our rest rooms. The doors had to be widened in some cases. Tension on doors had to be adjusted. Safety railings had to be installed inside restrooms. Since I was responsible for the expenses which directly affected profitability, I was against all these changes. I knew they had to be done, but I resisted in every way I could.

The ADA law raised my awareness about handicapped people in a negative way. I never saw one person in a wheel chair go into any of our stores. It seemed like such a waste of money for people who weren't going to ever use all the nice changes we made. I began to pay attention to handicap parking places in the community with much greater intent.

In the bigger retail stores, shopping centers, and movies there were way too many spots for "handicap only" vehicles. And, people who got out of the cars parked in them didn't seem have anything wrong with them. They walked just fine. No wheelchair, no cane, no squat. Of course, my bias at that time only allowed me to see what I wanted to see. The bigger picture was coming. I just didn't know it yet.

It seemed like most of the cars parked in the handicap parking were new and expensive. Most likely, they'd find the places where no car would bang into theirs and handicap slots were usually wider and had more room. I started looking at licenses and placards to see if they were legitimate. Usually, they were, but I got steamed when I saw one that wasn't.

I didn't have a clear and accurate perspective on handicapped people. I didn't really know anyone who was afflicted physically. I didn't have any relatives, neighbors, school buddies, or coworkers, past or present with physical impairments. I was totally in the dark about how they lived or what problems they had to face. But, it seemed like the new laws went over board to make a select few more comfortable.

The handicap bars on the walls in all the restrooms, adding ramps for sidewalk access, making entrance doors wider - it all hit as expenses on my profit and loss statements. The one on the wall to the side of the toilet at least made sense. Who would ever use the one on the wall behind the toilet any way?

Who's ever going to need them I asked myself? Why put something there no one will ever use? It seemed to me to be a clear cut example of government's power to force industry to spend their money unwisely.

I didn't see the money spent as having much benefit at all. I couldn't say that to anyone. I wouldn't tell somebody in a wheel chair how I felt. But, I never saw anyone I could talk to about it. I didn't see handicapped people buying gas. That was the only perspective I had.

Maybe most of them knew we pumped gas for them. Full service at self-service lanes. Another law. I didn't mind that one. It was not any extra cost, and it was a nice free service to offer. I had seen a few people take advantage of this. They sat there tying up a fuel lane and waited until some attendant came out, pumped their gas, collected the money or a credit card. That was good service. I believed in good service. True customer service was dying too fast in this country.

After a year and a half, taking two or three night courses each semester, I graduated with a 3.7 GPA at Florida Atlantic University. I earned my MPA (Masters in Public Administration), but I never used it. I enjoyed the classes, the fellowship of classmates and the challenges of working and going to school. My family gave me space and quiet time to do homework at home. I thought I would need the degree, but it never panned out. I had fun, enjoyed the intellectual challenges and neglected many of the day to day family needs. I now have two master's degrees. At least they will never be taken away from me.

One student there actually opened my eyes just a bit. He was a fellow grad student, but he was blind. I saw him come to campus, use elevators, use his walking stick to find his way down hallways and read Braille to know what room to go into. We never spoke, but I watched him carefully. He had to overcome obstacles unlike anything I had not ever encountered, nor probably ever would. And he did it every day. I admired him. I wish I had met him, but he was just another guy I saw on campus.

I had to move along and make the best use of my time. I had little time to socialize with students.

28

JANIS AND I had some serious talks about how we would spend the rest of our lives after Marysa and Weslee were gone, which wasn't too far off. Of all the things we liked to do, honestly, being around children and helping them grow up was what we liked to do best, so we decided to have two more kids. Alexandria was born the next year and two years later we had Janna.

I was there in the delivery room each time, just like the first two children except the technology had advanced a great deal and we could hear each baby's heart beat and watch meters flow on the delivery's progress. Janis was considered "high risk" but she made it through safely both times. I cried with both of my just born baby girls, just as I had done with Marysa and Weslee. There's no other experience that compares with watching the birth of your child. I wouldn't trade them for anything.

It seemed like all was going perfectly fine and then Texaco wanted me to move to Atlanta, Georgia. It was a lateral move, but I was being told that my position in Florida would soon end. So, I accepted it. It turned out they lied to me, and they filled my vacated position with someone else far less qualified. He had to transfer from Atlanta, from the same office I went to.

Janis was adamant. "I'm not moving! The kids are not moving." She wasn't going to move, nor were the kids. That was very clear. No room for negotiations there.

She explained her retirement years were worth too much to start all over again. It made sense. She had always moved for my career, now she had a big stake in her own.

"If you have to do it, do it. We'll come see you, or you can come see us. Take your pick. We can take turns once in a while. It's your job. Do what you have to do." I accepted the transfer.

I began commuting from Atlanta to Boca Raton, Florida, on Friday nights, returning to Atlanta Sunday nights. It was a 650 mile trip one way. I traveled 1300 miles each weekend.

I didn't adjust well from the get go. I lost a plane ticket. My Cross Texaco pen and pencil slipped out of my pockets. My gold money clip, given to me as a going away present from the members at Hillcrest Country Club got lost with several hundred dollar bills. A favorite Texaco watch disappeared.

After two months I ran out of moving benefits which paid for my plane tickets so I began driving my car home and back. Nine hours each way.

Not surprisingly, I made some errors at work. I had a hard time keeping track of a huge spreadsheet with market share numbers from half the US. I was accused of doing things I didn't do, but it wasn't a happy place for me to work. I endured it for nine months and quit. I missed my family. The job was not what I expected. There were a lot of changes imminent with Texaco and Shell merging. Many layoffs would be forthcoming soon. The handwriting was clearly embossed on the wall. Plus, I was really getting worn out, traveling and working long hours..

The long hours of driving lent itself the opportunity to think about my life, and gave me a chance to write poetry about it. When I had it worked out in my mind, I wrote it down.

HICHIN' TO ATLANTA

Hitchin' to Atlanta. You know the weather is fine.
Goin' to Atlanta in the summer.
Hitchin' to Atlanta. It's time to make some time.
Hitchin' to Atlanta on a weekend for two.

Pushin', Pushin'. Gotta make this baby go.
Pushin', Pushin', in the summer.
Goin' to Atlanta. You know I love you so.
Hitchin' to Atlanta on a weekend for two.

Gonna find a dance floor this evenin'
Find some place where I can kick off my shoes.
Gonna do some boogie with my baby.
I'm hitchin' to Atlanta on a weekend for two.

Trees are gettin' taller, the moon is goin' down.
Day is gettin' hotter, rig is cookin'.
Hills are gettin' steeper, we're gettin' close to town.
Hitchin' to Atlanta on a weekend for two.

Gonna find a place with some rhythm.
Gonna sing a song just for you.

Goin' to make some music with my baby.
Hitchin' to Atlanta on a weekend for two.

LONG DISTANCE LOVER

I'm your long distance lover, and I'm leaving you again.
I'll be missing your sweet kisses and be dreaming until then.
I hold you for the longest time. I hate to let you go.
I store the moment in my mind, like a rose beneath the snow.

And even though I leave you and don't see you for a while.
You are always with me, your laughter and your smile.
I miss you in the morning, I miss your gentle touch.
I miss you at the strangest times. I love you, oh, so much.

I'm your long distance lover, I won't see you until then.
As soon as I am out the door, can't wait to see you again.
Traveling through each lonely city, doing what I do best.
Finding you is natural like a bird flying to its nest.

Sometimes I know we try too hard. Then we start to doubt it.
Never seems to go away. Never should have allowed it.
Life is not a fairy tale, but what we have is true.
Patience is the hardest thing, but love will see it through.

It's good I get to see you and be with you then I can.
I love it when I come to you and feel that I'm your man.
Lying close beside you gives me time to rediscover.
As long as I keep up this life I'll be your long distance lover.

LONELY TRAVELER

I fear that I will never feel somehow more lonely than right now.
I ponder how it came to be. How could I leave my family?
Could I not see a better way? Can I make right the wrong today?
Compelling reasons made it so. To earn my wage I had to go.

With each brief trip it's crystal clear – I
want my family to be near!
I see them every chance I get. The stay's
too short, the needs unmet.
I can't deny I miss so much to see their
smiles and feel their touch.
I'm torn between two worlds apart, their
absence truly breaks my heart.

I lie awake, I cannot sleep. And when I do, it's not too deep.
Awaken often, sick and weak. When will
this torture reach its peak?
Enduring sadness lies within. I long for times which will begin
To stabilize this churning life, concatenates my work and wife.

Atlanta and Ft. Lauderdale – two destinations on the trail.
No matter if I drive or fly it hurts each time I say good-bye.
The common thread that holds my mind
is that I pray somehow to find
A way to stop this compromise, and soon before my own demise.

It is my one bright ray of hope, it gives me calming ways to cope.
I will prevail, my love's too strong to let this turmoil last too long.

Solutions often lay and hide, so close and yet so far and wide.

A different way to look and see, the

answer comes, and now I'm free.

29

AND THEN I had a chance for it to end.

"Come work for me and stop killing yourself." I knew Barry before the issue came up. He was my son-in-law's father. His offer was generous and it didn't take me but a few seconds to accept it. I began working for Memcorp, Inc. My commute immediately shortened from 9 hours one way to less than one hour one way.

As tired as I had felt those last months with Texaco I thought like maybe there were times when I was depressed, too, but I didn't know for sure. I have never felt depressed before and really didn't know how to recognize it. I was probably just tired, frustrated, and unfulfilled.

With two young girls to raise and not being certain of the future, I took on a second job working at a McDonald's restaurant. I was soon promoted to Swing Manager and closed the store Friday, Saturday and Sunday nights putting in about 22-25 hours per week.

I also started jogging again, something I did off and on over different times in my life. My neighborhood was quiet and lent itself well to running in the evening safely and without disturbing other people. I worked my way up to about 3 – 4 miles once or twice a week.

I looked forward to it. Jogging was a way to think and be alone with myself, and strengthen myself at the same time. I always stretched out before starting. I was always psyched up to get going and always ran until I couldn't go any further. No set distance, just as far as I could push myself.

"What is this? What's happening to me?"

One evening something strange happened. My left foot started dragging on the street and I couldn't keep it from catching and tripping me. I wasn't that tired. But, my left leg wouldn't stretch out as far forward as my right, and my left foot caught on the pavement. It was not happening to my right one, only my left foot. I nearly fell the first time it happened. I did fall the next time and scraped up both knees and both arms.

What's going on, I asked myself? What would make this happen like this? I was baffled.

Every time I ran, my left foot would start dragging long before I wanted to stop. No longer could I run until I was exhausted and I couldn't go any further. Now, I had to stop after about 2 miles, or I would trip. I just put up with it, and didn't give it much thought. I blamed it on my age. I had no clue this was a neurological issue and was a key factor identifying I had MS. Why didn't somebody tell me?

Janis noticed another change. "Stephen, look at you. You are gray. I don't want you to do that to yourself anymore. You look like you are dying. You need to cut out the running." She watched me walk in the door and flop onto the couch.

"You look pale. Half-dead. You look awful. This has got to stop."

I always ran until I couldn't go any further. I've always pushed myself to the max. This was different. My body wouldn't let me go the distance. My left leg seemed to be pooping out before my right leg. Maybe I was pushing it too much. Maybe my age was catching up in a strange way.

Of course, it was warm and humid outside, but in south Florida it's always warm and humid. I never got grey looking before. And, I used to run a lot farther. Something was different, wrong, amiss, screwy, puzzling. I had no answer. It had to be I was just getting older. But, my left leg was just as old as my right, so why was the left leg always the one that acted weaker?

My legs became stiff in a weird way. I couldn't walk normally after running. My legs felt swollen and like logs. I waddled precariously into the family room turned and fell backwards onto the couch. Now every time I jogged that was how it ended. A repeat performance. Ditto. It was predictable. I thought maybe I needed to stretch more before going out for the run. I usually stretched about 5 minutes. I tried stretching ten minutes, but it didn't help.

Stretching my legs longer before jogging yielded the same results, the left leg wouldn't keep up with the right one after about two miles.

I finally accepted it as a function of age. It never crossed my mind there was a neurological problem at work. Why should I? I'd been healthy all my life, and I was still healthy.

Another thing that had been happening for a while – I continually had black and blue toes. I started having two or three going at any one time. I stubbed my toes a lot and they took the brunt of my suddenly clumsy feet. Just some dried blood under the nail. But, it took a long time to grow out and start anew. Sometimes I kicked something I didn't know was there, or I ran into a chair or wall I was trying to go around and just made a tiny wrong step. The worst was when I caught a toe on the carpet and bent it backwards. I could feel it and hear my toe go "pop!" It happened walking and also going up, and going down stairs at the house. I used to sprain fingers as a kid playing basketball, but toes, never. This was different than when I was younger, but I am causing harm to myself.

I started blaming Janis for my beat up toes. Every time I kicked a chair out of place or a hit a book on the floor or kicked a bag by the door I blamed Janis. After all, I was still the same old me. Why I was suddenly so spastic had to be because things were in my way. Things I didn't put there and didn't know to look out for them.

It never once occurred to me that my clumsy feet, my black and blue toes and the problems I had with my left foot when jogging could be related. Why should I? There was nothing wrong with me.

30

MANAGING A MCDONALDS had a few fringe benefits. I got to eat free, and so did my family. Janis would bring the girls to see me and we would have dinner together if it wasn't too busy. I ate plenty of cheeseburgers and French fries. I usually ate again while I was closing up. I never gained weight because I was working and jogging and burning it all off. I also drank a lot of coffee. Always with Half and Half cream and Sweet and Low.

I had had a perfect safety record at work for all the years I had been employed, not counting my mishaps in my younger years on the golf course in high school or when I was working the grain elevator. The chemical plant in Houston had been the most dangerous environment in my career but, I was a safe employee there and learned many valuable lessons working for a safety-conscious corporation. With Phillips and Texaco I had averaged driving 30,000-40,000 miles a year without one accident. I was always walking around garage bays, convenience stores, and busy gas islands. I was vigilant of potentially dangerous situations. I've preached safety with my employees, and it had been a priority I never ignored.

One late afternoon at my full time job my company's store room was low on copy paper and I went to buy a few cases. I lifted them out of my car and onto the loading dock. A gray metal gate stood on the foot of the dock and blocked people from entering, but also allowed breeze to pass through its strong braided iron mesh. The gate was made of heavy gage steel and it weighed over 200 pounds.

Somehow I pushed one of the cases into the gate and it flipped up and over the edge and, BAM! As it flew out of control it whacked me across my forehead.

I could feel the steel bar as it ripped into the flesh in my skull and it knocked me down to the pavement below the dock. I lay still for a few seconds wondering how badly I had been hit, and how bad it was going to get. The blood started dripping freely. It flowed in response to each heart beat which was resonating loudly in my head every few seconds.

I realized no one knew where I was.

"Help! Help!" I screamed.

Soon Earl Smith walked over the edge of the dock and peered down at me.

"Oh, my God. Are you OK? What happened?"

I didn't move. I was afraid to. Something told me just to lie still.

"Something hit me in the head, Earl."

"Yeah, I see that big gate right beside you. You're lucky you're alive if that thing hit you. Stay there. We'll get help for you." He asked someone to call 911.

In a few minutes the ambulance came and two strong men lifted me onto a stretcher and carried me into their red emergency truck.

This was an all time first for me. I'd never been in an ambulance before. I'd never been "the injured party."

They asked me a few questions about how it happened, and measured my vital signs. I talked to them as they tried to stop the bleeding.

As soon as I arrived at the emergency room I was treated like a king. It was a new Cleveland Clinic Hospital that had just opened and business hadn't picked up yet, which was good for me. I had about 20 trained medical people standing there ready to help me. I was the only patient they had.

I got 14 stitches, just above the hairline over my left eye. They said it was just a routine cut, not too deep, and would heal in time. That was the hardest hit that I have ever felt to my head. My hard head came through again. I was going to be OK.

Thinking back, I survived it when GrandDaddy Weiss dropped me on a brass wastebasket when I was two. And the time Paul Kiser's swing hit me in first grade. I went unconscious in the ninth grade playing football. Chris Coyle barely missed my eye swinging his 2-iron, and I hit myself in the head with a crow bar at the grain elevator. And, under the influence of a drug I smashed my head into the floor in college. My head had been traumatized numerous times through the years, But, I was once again OK. I always got through it, never thinking once there might have been damage inside the brain tissues.

I started getting headaches more often. No problem. Just popped three aspirin in my mouth and twenty minutes later the headache was gone. But, they began happening more frequently, they became stronger, and sometimes aspirin did not make them go away. My head hurt in different places on different days. One day it would ache in the back of my neck. The next night it would hurt in my forehead. Another time I felt pain only on the right side of my head.

I decided to see a neurologist to see what was causing all these headaches. Janis agreed. My family doctor, Dr. Patrick Mulhern, referred me to a local neurologist. Janis was acutely aware of changes in my behavior as well, but I wasn't. It was time for answers. She thought I was becoming more unreasonable, less logical, less patient.

LIFE AFTER DIAGNOSIS

31

I WALKED INTO his office and it was a warm busy atmosphere. Lots of people bustling about. I read the doctor's credentials, at least the big print, displayed in large black frames on the wall. Graduated medical school New York, 1953. Graduated in Neurology 1955 somewhere in New Jersey. He had won many awards and been recognized for many achievements, but I expected him to be rather old. He was. I saw him talking to another patient and laughing about something. I finished filling out all the insurance forms and waited.

I was called into a room and sat on the side of a bed. He walked up to me.

"Mr. Knapp I'm Dr. Bernstein. Tell me why you are here."

"Hi. I've been getting too many headaches. I'd like to know why."

Over the next twenty minutes he checked my eyes, and my ears. He asked lots of questions about my health and family history while he banged a rubber hammer on each of my knee caps. He wrote a prescription for Amnytriptylene for my headaches. When he was finished he told me to get an MRI and gave me directions where to get it. He said nothing about what I might have, or what was causing the headaches. I guessed he needed the MRI to be certain.

I arrived at the MRI office and there was only one lady there who gave me more paperwork I was directed to a room where I took off everything metal – watch, belt, coins, car keys. She showed me a locker with a key. She kept the key but promised to return it when we were done. Then we walked into a bare, stark room with a funny looking machine in the middle facing the door.

It was very quiet in the room and rather sterile. No pictures, no plants, no music, no magazines. There was just an imposing round machine with smooth edges.

"This is our MRI machine – magnetic resonance imaging. Have you ever had one before?"

I indicated I had not.

"It's completely safe. You won't feel a thing. You just lie here and be still." She gestured for me to lie down and then she pushed a button and I slid horizontally into a round doughnut looking structure. She gave me headphones before I entered it.

"What kind of music do you like?"

"Huh?"

"Rock and roll, classical, jazz? The music drowns out some of the noise made by the machine."

"Oh. Rock and roll, I guess."

"OK. This will take about 45 minutes. The main thing is to lie still and don't move."

She moved me automatically further into the machine. My head had a round curved surface over me. I wore the head phones. It got so quiet it was spooky.

"Are you OK in there?" She was talking to me from another room.

"Yeah. Fine. Sure. I'm ready to go. Let it rip." I had no idea what to expect but it would start very soon.

"I Want to Hold Your Hand" by the Beatles started playing and soon after a low tone, sort of like an electric piano out of tune, or a tug boat stuck in first gear, sounded for a few seconds. That song always reminded me of being in Coffeyville in the 60's, working at KGGF, playing records like that one on the radio.

Every so often it would bleep for a few seconds and then stop. On. Off. On. Off. The music really didn't drown it out at all, but I guess it would have been more annoying without the music. Then it was over. No big deal.

A few days later I returned to Dr. Bernstein. "I see something, actually two somethings, but I'm not sure," he told me. "Let's see what happens in three months and we'll have you try another MRI." I made an appointment for three months later and walked out.

I started writing poetry more often. It was always something I enjoyed once in a while, and I had been writing a poem every Christmas since the year after we were married called the Knapp Recap which we sent to all our friends with holiday cards. However, my creative juices seemed to be stronger and quite often riding to work or back an idea and words would come to me and I would write them down.

As the months rolled by a few things became clear. I was still having headaches. The Amnytriptylene had no effect. Much later I would learn the medication was for depression, not headaches. My jogging was still being interrupted by my left foot. I was wondering what the two "things" were he saw on the MRI and what would he see the next time around?

The second MRI proved to be exactly like the first in the way it still showed two things, whatever those were. Dr. Bernstein had a short meeting with me after reviewing the results of the second MRI.

"Well, Stephen. You have two lesions. They seem to be getting worse. You have MS – the Multiple Sclerosis."

I listened but I didn't know how to react to this news.

And then he really shocked me. "There is nothing that I can do for it. So, don't come back. There is nothing I can do. Oh, if you can, try and get some insurance for it. Good luck. Bye." We shook hands and I walked out his door confused and bewildered. I didn't know whether to thank him or strangle him. I had to go home and read about MS first.

I tried to get some disability insurance, but there were some problems. I had to answer a very detailed questionnaire and had to list the medication and the MRI's. I never got the insurance approved. The doctor wasn't very savvy on insurance requisites and their policies. Once I filled the prescription, and had the first MRI any chance of getting insurance was doomed. Red flags could not be ignored I had something very wrong with me and no insurance company would take the risk.

32

I BEGAN TO research Multiple Sclerosis. I read some books. I read some articles on the internet. I didn't really get it. I didn't feel like I had anything unusual. The information I read didn't seem to apply to me. I wasn't showing symptoms of optic neuritis. I wasn't having paralysis. There were no exacerbations. I had no evidence of shaking, nothing I read applied to me. After I felt I had a handle on what MS was, I didn't really believe the doctor. Not me. No way. I was just fine. I was as OK as always.

I took the family to attend an MS seminar in Miami. A doctor showed slides about what MS was and how it affected the brain and the central nervous system. Then a woman with MS made an excellent and memorable presentation. She was the CEO of a family business and one day she just woke up blind and partially paralyzed. In a few months she had recovered, but was still bothered by symptoms and had "good and bad days."

She looked normal. She had been a model earlier in her career and was still very attractive. Her story did not fit with my understanding of MS. It was my first real glimpse that you could have all kinds of internal symptoms that no one could see, and look perfectly normal and healthy on the outside. I began changing my thinking about what MS was. She said she personified the expression, "But, you look so good," often spoken to a person with MS. It was certainly true of her. If she hadn't told us she had MS I would have never known.

Janis talked to me about her later that day. "Steve, you should get a second opinion. There has to be more that we can do." She found a neurologist with MS patients and I went through the whole thing again. Forms, physical exam, MRI, but this one had a few more enlightening tidbits to share with me.

I had saved my last MRI and we compared it to the one I just took. They were well back lit, side by side, and one set of pictures, the most recent set, clearly had more white inflammation than the other one. Janis and I both waited to hear what Dr. Nunez, my new neurologist, had to say.

"These are lesions," she pointed to the white shapeless images. "There are more lesions now than three months ago. You are a walking time bomb about to explode at any moment! I can't believe you don't have the usual array of MS symptoms, but the evidence is here." She tapped her fingers at the MRI. "It's just a matter of time."

"Are you sure?" I was still in disbelief. Walking time bomb. No way.

I was skeptical. I thought back to the days I was in the fairways at Coffeyville Country Club watching the sky grow dark on the horizon. I could estimate with pin point accuracy if it would rain or not. This was different. I didn't know anything about lesions, or MRI's or Multiple Sclerosis. I really did not know what to expect. "A walking time bomb" got my attention, and Janis's, but when were the fireworks going to start? She couldn't tell me that.

Dr. Nunez responded by mentioning two more tests – a spinal tap and an evoked potential test. "Once we get the results back from them we will have a much better idea if you have MS."

"We can do the spinal tap now if you have time. I'll have to schedule the other one next week."

"Sure. OK." I was not apprehensive at all. I hoped maybe she'd find something to disprove her original diagnosis. I had read that an MRI by itself might not necessarily be conclusive. I wanted to be absolutely sure. If that meant more tests, that was fine with me.

I was moved into a small room with a bed, took off my shirt and put on a hospital gown. Then I was instructed to lie sideways on the bed with my back facing the wall.

"This doesn't hurt at all," she told me. She put a needle into me to anesthetize any pain I might have felt. The doctor stood behind me with four empty glass tubes and started filling fluid into each, one at a time, and handed them to her assistant. I felt like I was maple tree being drained of its syrup. My clear liquid spinal fluid flowed rather quickly into the flasks and she was done in about 15 minutes. She was right. I couldn't feel a thing the whole time.

"Go home and lie down. You'll feel fine tomorrow." The doctor smiled. Janis and I walked out after making an appointment for the other test.

There was still doubt in my mind as to my diagnosis, even though the MRI seemed to indicate MS was what I had. Dr. Nunez told me the spinal tap was necessary for confirmation. It had been painless and I had never had one before. I thought it would be worth it to go one step more to bring closure to my wondering.

I did not know what I was about to go through, although a few others that I have talked to since then have had a similar painful experience that I was about to have. Further research and attending of more seminars has revealed mine was not unique, but it was to me.

In my subsequent research I have read about a few stories where people said their spinal tap was painful in its aftermath. I presumed as MS is different with each person, so are the reactions to diagnostics. I was naïve, but hopeful that the spinal tap, or lumbar puncture, or LP as it is also called, would shed more light on my diagnosis. The spinal tap took place on a Thursday afternoon.

I sat on the couch at home and felt very normal except for a mild headache. Headaches were common for me, so I was thinking this procedure was done and I had made it though with no problems. I went to work the next morning but my headache intensified, and by noon I left the office and went to bed. On a scale of 1 to 10, my headache had risen to about an 8, and I was very much in pain and discomfort. I lay in bed watching TV wondering when the pain would subside. I was taking 3 Advils every 3 hours, but the pain persisted with no improvement.

I called the doctor to see if she could prescribe something stronger for the pain, but she was away and I had to call her backup. I left a message to call me. Slowly, it occurred to me that my doctor had told me to lie flat, which I had not been doing, so I tossed the pillow on the floor, and there was a mild improvement, although the pain had increased to a higher level. When I got up to go the bathroom, or to eat something, the pain surged. It was now at 10 on my hypothetical scale. It was more painful than any headache I had ever known.

I have had a lot of headaches in my life, but never one like this. The pain was from ear to ear, from the top of my head to the bottom of my neck. My whole head was in pain and it had become more than just uncomfortable.

Friday night I did not sleep much as the pain was too great. Any slight movement made it worse. I must have had many short periods of sleep filled with dreams that I could remember upon wakening, but the clock by the bed moved ever so slowly through the night.

Saturday morning came with no relief. I called the back-up doctor again and left an urgent message, I needed help now. I laid in bed, flat, not wanting to eat, move, or talk. I just wanted the pain to go away. It was then that I realized what was going on.

The spinal fluid circulates through the brain and the spinal cord. It serves as a buffer between the brain and the skull. I was feeling pressure caused by the absence of the fluid. It was as if my head was in a giant vice, screwed tightly against it, which is why I felt the pain all over everywhere in my head. As the day progressed the pain increased to a level that was getting hard to take, but there was no escape. I couldn't sleep. It was too painful to sit up. I did not want to drink much, because I knew I would have to relieve myself more often if I loaded up on liquids. It became unbelievable conscious endurance. More like torture. I had to modify my made-up scale. This was now up to about 20.

I have never felt pain like this. It is beyond anything I had ever known.

I did not sleep Saturday night until about 4 am. Pure exhaustion took over and spared some compassion. I woke up about 7 am, feeling as tired and as much in pain as the night before. There still was no word from the doctor. Every movement increased an already high degree of pain. I was in bed, motionless with no pillow, feeling hopeless. I felt like I was not going be able to handle this pain much longer. Saturday spilled into Sunday, but it was just more endless endurance. My whole head was in constant pain. I started thinking how I could terminate this pain. I wanted to die if that what it took to stop the pain.

Suicide is something I had never seriously considered before, but I was thinking about it then. How could I do it? Where? What could I do to get ready for it? Obviously, the pain was not going to go away, the doctor was not going to call, and I couldn't wait any longer. It was beyond intolerable. It had been intolerable for too long and my patience, my fortitude, my hope, my will – they were all used up.

Monday I was in the house by myself. My wife was at work, and my children were at school. It was time to take action and put my pain to rest. My only problem was that I was upstairs and everything I might need was downstairs. Knives were in the kitchen. I could slit my wrists. The pool was outside. I could drown myself. The car was in the driveway. I could drive into a canal or hit a wall. I had numerous plans. I only had to do one of them, but it was too painful to go down the stairs.

I was contemplating how I was going to do it when the phone rang. It was the back-up doctor. I told him how much pain I was in, and that I had had a spinal tap Thursday. He advised me to stay flat until my body had regenerated the fluid in my Central Nervous System. He called in the prescription. I lay in bed praying my wife would be home soon, so that she could get the painkillers that I desperately needed. My hope that an end to the pain was close had been restored. I figured I had made it that far. I could wait a few more hours.

What I took was called Butalbital. It helped a great deal, but not completely. I was still in pain, although, thankfully, to a lesser degree, and my previous thoughts had been forever erased. Monday evening my wife called my son in Atlanta, who checked the internet and said I should be drinking coffee for the pain. It worked! Tuesday I went to work pain free.

From Thursday afternoon to Monday evening, over four days in time, I was in a kind of pain that I have never, ever experienced. It was a type of headache pain that filled the entire head. It was relentless. It was excruciating. And it was all for a test just to confirm that I had MS. If I had to do it again, I would not do it. It may not have been the norm, as no one I have talked to who had a spinal tap had an experience this severe. But, I would not wish this experience on my worst enemy. It was absolutely horrible.

33

LATER THAT WEEK Dr. Nunez called to say I had MS. The spinal tap cinched it. But she still wanted to do the evoked potential test as further confirmation. I acquiesced. Surely it wouldn't be as painful and horrendous as what I just went through.

I learned that evoked potential tests measure electrical activity in certain areas of the brain in response to stimulation of certain groups of nerves. These tests are often used to assist in the diagnosis of MS because they can indicate problems along the pathways of certain nerves that are too subtle to be noticed or found on a doctor's exam. Problems along the nerve pathways are a direct result of the disease. The demyelination caused the nerve impulses to be slowed, garbled, or halted altogether.

I read there were three main types of evoked potential tests:

Visual Evoked Potentials (VEP): You sit in front of a screen on which an alternating checkerboard pattern is displayed. Brainstem Auditory Evoked Potentials (BAEP): You hear a series of clicks in each ear.

Sensory Evoked Potentials (SEP): Short electrical impulses are administered to an arm or leg.

My tests were the third kind. It took about 2 ½ hours. There were many different parts of my arm and legs to test. Each segment took some set up time as the tester attached tiny wires to my skin. There was no pain, and very little discomfort, during the tests. Each test produced a graph. There was a feeling of being shocked but they were mild enough I could handle them.

I kept telling myself this was so much better than the spinal tap. I watched the graph drive a pen up and down squiggling lines. I could easily match the shocks with blips and spikes on the graph, but I really didn't know how to interpret the markings or patterns. The two ladies who were giving me the tests were not allowed to comment.

They gave me a sort of a disclaimer talking about how only a qualified certified medical professional was allowed to discuss the charts. Maybe they just didn't know. Later my neuro told me nothing was out of the expected range, and she held firm on her diagnosis.

Welcome to the world of MS, Stevo. I still did not know how to react to this confusing, contradicting news. I should have felt like I had MS, and I patently did not. Even if I didn't know what it was supposed to feel like, I was skeptical. I've always felt normal. I was still normal. No matter how many lesions I had. I was no different than the Stephen Knapp I had always known myself to be.

Dr. Nunez's words – "You are a walking time bomb about to explode at any moment!" I played that quote over and over in my mind wondering when and if the explosion would start. I could hear her words, but the reality was I was still in disbelief.

Maybe it already had started and I just didn't know it. It was confusing.

When my diagnosis was confirmed my neurologist gave me three pamphlets. Rebif had not been put on the market yet. I read about Avonex, Betaseron and Copaxone. Even after studying the material I was not 100% sure about what I was going to do. She told me to choose one because I had to be happy with it, and I was the one who was going to be taking it, so the choice was mine. She told me they were all good. They all worked successfully in most cases. They all were approved by FDA, and supported with clinical trials that slowed the disease's progression and protracted the time between attacks. They all required being administered by taking a shot.

My only reservations were two-fold – 1. They all had been FDA approved for Relapse Remitting Multiple Sclerosis, and 2. I probably had never had an RRMS attack. I wondered if I should be taking medication for something not designed for what I had. I was of the belief that if I had MS, then I had Primary Progressive MS, but it would take more time to determine if that was the case. Nunez wouldn't say what type I had. There was no FDA approved medication for Primary Progressive MS. There were not many ways to get an objective determination of whether PPMS is getting better or worse, or staying the same, since attacks, or exacerbations, were not part of my equation. I found out it took years of building a history to know for sure. My history wasn't that long yet. My MS records were just beginning.

I considered one of the differences between medications was how often each was taken – Avonex was once a week, Betaseron was every other day, and Copaxone was every day. Nonetheless, she wrote a prescription for Betaseron, which is the one I had chosen. She said it was a good choice, it was the strongest medicine of all of them.

I am not paid to promote this product, but having taken it for over 5 years (as of this writing), I am happy with my decision. Originally, I chose it on the basis of its being in the middle. One had to be taken daily, the other was once a week. My choice was every other day. Given that they all worked then this was a middle of the road kind of choice. It also had the strongest single dosage which appealed to me.

That was an all-time first. All my life the doctor, what ever doctor I had at the time, had written my prescriptions for me to take without discussion of choice, unless I was allergic to it. I also liked it when a nurse came to my house and taught me how to take it, while the rest of my family watched.

October 27, 2002, the Betaseron nurse knocked on our door. It was a thorough but personal and comfortable lesson, given in the comfort of my home. Since that day there have been some follow-up calls to me to see how I was doing on the medication. It is a standard service, but it was nice to know I am not forgotten, and can ask questions 24-7 if I have any concerns.

The side effects lasted about three months and that was not a pleasurable time. Looking back on it, I can understand why some people give up on taking medication, or switch, looking for a better, more effective and more friendly, one. I will never know how much my MS was affecting me, and how much the medication was affecting me, and probably it was a combination of both.

I had feverish days. I had aches and pains all over my body. I felt like I had the flu. I felt nauseous. I lacked energy. I had trouble sleeping. And I had headaches. I began taking aspirin before and after each shot, which helped a little bit. All in all, it was basically three months of feeling sick. Nothing has ever compared with how long it lasted. I have had my share of flu bugs, but never one that lasted three months. They were all classic symptoms, predicted in the Betaseron literature, predicted by the nurse. I reasoned the short-term discomfort was a necessary evil, but offset by longer term gains which I would not receive if I didn't go through with taking it regularly.

I put up with it on the hope it would only last for three months and I was doing the right thing in taking it. On the one hand, I tend to be a naturalist, and I don't like foreign substances going into my body. On the other hand, reading the results of the clinical trials, I was improving my chances by taking it, which overturned my initial urges not to take anything.

I joined the local MS chapter and began getting a flood of information, most of which made little sense to me since I still had no MS symptoms. Little did I know or even suspect that my symptoms were there. They had been there for years, and they were growing. However, they were simply invisible to me. I admit I was also blind as to what I was looking for.

34

I JOINED A local MS Chapter and that put me on several mailing lists. My family and I were invited to join a select group of families all of which had a family member dealing with MS. It was called a retreat and we spent a weekend at a remote location far from the hustle and bustle of the customary chaotic life we were living in.

It was an awesome experience for all of us. I can best describe it by sharing a thank you letter I wrote after we had returned home.

"It was the humble pleasure of my family to enjoy the awesome experience this weekend, 1/23-1/26/03, of the Family Retreat Weekend and the Elk's Camp, for the selected families that are dealing with Multiple Sclerosis. It was an exceptional weekend that we will all treasure for the rest of our lives. To say "Thank you" seems hardly enough, but I wanted to express our deepest appreciation to all who were involved.

It is impossible to pinpoint one shining moment that stands above the rest because there were so many positive components to the event. I am still absorbing and enjoying them in reflection. My children met other children who face the same questions and uncertainties, and they all bonded together so well and really had a lot of fun together. The "care takers" met as a group and were advised on common issues that helped them to understand MS better and develop new coping skills. Those of us who have MS got the chance to speak freely to each other about our personal stories of pain, suffering, being misunderstood, being mis-diagnosed, and maybe, for the first time in our lives, being understood by those among us who have felt exactly the same feelings. It was very powerful. It was very good. We came together as strangers, and left as more than just as friends. We all had a common set of characteristics that only we, and others like us, can share. There is inestimable value in the comfort of knowing that there are others just like us, and that we are not alone. It is something that even our spouses and children cannot fully appreciate.

The energy of the staff and volunteers added greatly to the enjoyment of the weekend. I have never been to an event where I felt like the volunteers were in greater numbers than the guests. It was incredible. Everyone was so helpful, so friendly, so willing to do whatever was needed. They were "The Dream Team!" We could not have been treated better. For so many to sacrifice their weekend for us is truly appreciated, and please convey our thanks to all of them for all of their efforts. They made our weekend very special.

In closing, on behalf of my family, my new friends, and myself, thank you for giving us a rare opportunity. We came together from different walks of life, different races, different educational and financial backgrounds and we shared something so precious that we will never be the same again. We all grew together as a group with mutual respect and understanding. We grew as individuals, learning more about ourselves and learning from the professionals who were there to answer our questions. Altogether, it was a great weekend for everyone that took part. Thanks so very much.

Sincerely,

Stephen F. Knapp"

This gathering left a profound impression on me and my understanding of MS. It was my first time being around a group who all had the same disease. My first thoughts were pity. My second thoughts were a conviction that somehow I would not allow myself to be like them. I would fight as hard as I could to maintain my health, at least more so than what I saw in this group.

They were all worse than I was. Some of them were much worse. Several women arrived in wheelchairs or electric powered scooters. Others had different kinds of types of assistive walking devices. They had suffered from MS much longer than I had. They were more experienced in coping with it than I was. I could never picture myself having that much difficulty. I was still jogging. I felt guilty. I wasn't going to mention the jogging. Initially, I did not see we had much in common, but, I knew I could learn volumes from them.

"All right. Everyone listen up. I want the MSers to sit in a circle in this room. I want the caretakers to follow Dr. Schwartz into that room. All the children go with Katy outside for games. If any children want to stay with their parent, it's OK, but you have to be real quiet."

Dr. Schwartz spoke candidly to the caretakers. I didn't hear him but Janis filled me in. He talked about how people with MS were trying to cope with their weaknesses, their insecurities and the changes in their bodies and minds. He said to expect them to lie, to be lazy, sneak around to hide things. He said they would pull hard against the good nature of the caretaker and cause the caretaker to get sick, worn out and feel helpless and unappreciated. As the MS patient loses their job, their ability to help around the house, and to do the things they used to do the caretaker has to take up the slack – the void created by the MS patient's inability to perform as they once did. The burden falls directly on the caretaker by default, not by choice or democratic process. Bottom line – he said it's not any easy job being a caretaker.

In our own room out of earshot from that group, we had a Doctor of Psychiatry sit with us. She admitted she did not know much about MS, but that wasn't important. She gave us the stage. One at a time we went around the circle and spoke about our MS, and how it affected our families, our jobs, our marriages and whatever else we wanted to add. Everyone had a sob story except me. Every person's story was different, and some were real tearjerkers.

Bess lost her husband to divorce. She lost her job that she loved. She couldn't do the work any longer. Her memory was going and she couldn't type anymore because she had no feeling in her fingers. She lost her children along with the divorce because she couldn't support them. She lost her house, her friends, her neighbors, and if that wasn't enough, she lost her confidence, and her self esteem. She lost all semblance of hope of ever having happiness again. Her mother took care of her, but her mother was getting too old to be very helpful. She had no idea who would care for her in a few more years when her mother was no longer capable of helping her. Meanwhile, her insurance had long ago stopped paying for her medications and she was nearly broke.

Jane lost two husbands and two families before she realized she had MS. She had been diagnosed with several different other maladies and had spent thousands of dollars on medications and doctor visits and treatments that did not make her feel better. She was all alone and poor. She had lost her vision in her right eye for a while, but it came back. Another time she was paralyzed on her right side and couldn't walk. But, then that went away. Several doctors had told her it was all in her head and there was nothing physically wrong with her. She thought she was crazy.

Shelly lived with her mother. She was diagnosed at 16. He mother became her full time caretaker, who pulled away from her husband who couldn't handle it. So, Shelly and her mother lived together in a small apartment on government money. They were resigned to accept it was just them for the rest of their lives, and she was worried what would happen when her mother passed away.

Joan lost a baby through a miscarriage and then she was told by her doctor she should not have any more because the medication was too much and not safe enough for her to try to get pregnant. She had us all teary-eyed about how she wanted to have another child. She was in a wheel chair too weak to even speak out very strongly. It was without saying she could not bear another child just looking at her.

Sharon used to be an executive for a big corporation. She had to step down because she couldn't keep up with the pressure. Her memory was failing her and she made too many errors, not accepted in her level of authority. Her ability to multitask became too limited. She couldn't do her job anymore. She had had several exacerbations which came at crucial times professionally when she couldn't respond to her responsibilities. She had lost a husband in the changes because he couldn't understand and or accept her as a less than healthy productive person. He couldn't accept his new role as a caretaker which was what she needed, so he left her. She went through severe depression. It was only after she had lost most of that which was important to her that she learned that she had MS.

Joanne had been diagnosed with about five different diseases and took thousands of dollars in medications, and several operations, which didn't help. Every time she had an attack a different doctor gave her a different story about what was causing it. One doctors told her it was just in her head. She had been mis-diagnosed over and over and thought she was the only one who had what she had. She thought it must be so rare nobody knew about it.

It went on and on. Sadness, despair, losses, pain – both physical and mental. Financial loss, relationships lost. It was hard to take, and I was just listening. They were living their stories. When it was my turn, I praised everyone for their courage. I was feeling the electric tingling sensations in my legs during my talk. I had only felt them a few times before then. I mentioned the sensations to the group and told them my story didn't have the severity of the ones who had already poured their hearts out to us. I didn't have anything similar to pour out about my life.

I was the only male in the group. There were 12 females with MS and me. It was in the group setting that I learned the ratio of women versus men with MS was about 3 to 1, women being the larger percentage. I talked about losing a career in the Air Force, and I was new to MS, so I hadn't had the range of experiences the others had had to face.

When we ended the session I was the only one who just got up and walked away. Everyone else needed some help. I wondered if I would ever get to be like them. If I would ever face the kinds of anguish and hardship and sorrow I heard that day. I wondered if I would ever get fired or lose my family. Would I ever not be able to walk? These were sobering thoughts I could not answer, and hoped I would never have to.

35

ONE MORNING AFTER returning to work I entered the building and was talking to Robert, who was in charge of our accounting department. "Robert, I need to go to the building next door and I'd like you to join me. I have a few questions…." Whap!

"Are you OK?" Robert looked at my body sprawled spread eagle on the floor. The mail I had in my left hand flew all over. The keys I had in my right hand felt like they had permanently indented grooves in my palm. I was flushed, embarrassed, and got up awkwardly.

My foot caught on the floor and I lost my balance. Simple as that. But, it was totally unexpected. I recovered. I wasn't really hurt. Just shocked that it happened.

Robert helped me gather my mail and offered," Are you sure you are OK?"

"No problem. Just a little clumsy, that's all."

Only a few days later I was at the Post Office walking in the parking lot toward the building. Thud! "Arrggh."

My left foot had caught on the curb and I fell forward. I landed on my hands and knees. Two people rushed to see if I was all right. I bounced right but up and warded them off.

"Thanks. I'm OK. No reason to worry."

My daughter, Marysa mentioned it to me. "Dad. Something is wrong. Your gait is different. What's going on? What's wrong?"

I didn't tell her. I dodged her question. I wasn't ready to tell anyone, yet.

A few days later the scratched and bruises showed on my knees and palms, but in time I healed completely. I thought it was weird that I had lifted up my foot unconsciously over that same curb for years without ever stumbling. I figured I must be getting stiff and needed to stretch more in the morning. It must have been just an age thing.

"You are a walking time bomb about to explode at any moment!" I wondered if these were the early signs of things to come? No. Not yet, I decided. It would have to be more than that, surely.

Denial was something I embraced daily for many months until I started walking so awkwardly I had to let the truth out. I fell 6 times in about 2 months and that was also a reason for letting people know what I had. But, even then it hadn't sunk in completely until I applied for handicap parking, which I was still reluctant to do. Dr. Nunez wrote, "Stephen Knapp has Multiple Sclerosis and is permanently disabled" on the form.

When I read those words a new sense of acceptance came over me. It was really real. I was still stunned by it. Do you know what I mean? You know but you don't want to believe it, and then you do. With me there was a big hiatus between the announcement of the diagnosis and the moment I fully accepted the reality of what the diagnosis meant. But, also, it was all about being able to tell other people candidly that I had MS. Doing that is what made it acceptable to me. I could not believe it as long as I could hide it, but when I had to admit it to others, I had to admit it to myself first. The words -"I have MS," was hard to say. I had to get past my own resistance. In time, it became easier to say, but it did not come without lots of time, and many struggles.

36

THE PROBLEM WITH being in denial is that you have to step away from yourself, or rely on someone else whose opinion you trust to know that you are in a world of disbelief. You can't see it, or taste it, or feel it, or smell it. Acknowledgement did not come easily or all at once.

Because MS affected me in so many different ways, it was easy to fall into the trap of rationalization for each of them. As I moved from mostly migraines, to a myriad of MS related symptoms, I slipped into very irrational justifications for both what I was feeling and how the MS was impacting me.

After my initial diagnosis I continued to jog, as I had done off and on for years past, but could not understand why my left foot dragged on the pavement after a few laps around the block. I wasn't tired yet, and felt I could have run much further, but I had to stop or risk tripping or falling. Why was this happening? I hadn't yet connected the dots between my foot catching while jogging and falling on the curb.

My neurologist explained that it was not so much that my legs had gotten weaker, but rather that the Central Nervous System's

(CNS) signals had been "short circuited" when sent to my legs. The lesions in my brain showed clear evidence that some inflammation and demylination was disturbing the nerves in my leg.

My own reasoning was that if I used the leg muscles it will help to keep them stronger than if I didn't use them at all. Therefore, I walked and exercised my legs daily even though I experienced various levels of pain, fatigue and weakness. I would only get worse, maybe sooner, if I stopped using my legs. The fear of losing total ambulation was a primary motivator for me. I couldn't see myself not ever walking again. It could happen, but I was committed to not letting it happen. I would fight my MS with exercise.

I decided if I ever got to the point where I was not able to walk safely then I would use mechanized means to move about, but I firmly believed the longer I could keep my legs strong, the longer I would be able to walk. To not use my legs at all when I could use them was inviting the time when I would be unable to walk on my own. That was a long way off, I hoped, and I vowed I would continue to push it further into the future. Despite the common thought that I should "take it easy" and not over do it, I believed just the opposite. I would only get worse unless I did push myself.

My quitting smoking in 1979, when I was 30 years old, had some similarities with what I was now facing. I didn't conquer one habit. I conquered about 50, one at a time. I used to light up first thing in the morning as I rolled down the window heading out the driveway to work. I usually smoked a second pulling into a parking space at work. I had my third cigarette with my first cup of coffee. If I had three cups of coffee in the morning, then I had three cigarettes as well.

My job at the country club afforded me the luxury of having as many Cokes as I wanted, and by midmorning I switched from coffee to Coke. The cold liquid seemed to sooth my dry throat. So, I had a couple of Cokes and had several cigarettes with each cup. Then, I had to have that last cigarette before lunch, and the next one right after lunch. Anything that was tense, that I needed to make a decision about, or ponder about, prompted me to need a smoke. Back and forth, smoke – drink – smoke – drink – eat – smoke – drink….. Each time I lit up was a different situation. I had to deal with each one of them. I had to break a different habit each time I faced each one of them.

MS was kind of like that. Each feeling was new and I had to adjust to it, one at a time.

As the tingly sensations began to increase in their frequency and intensity, both in my legs and in my arms and hands, I continued to assume that they were temporary aberrations. They did not hurt and were fascinating, for a while. Everyone knows what hitting your elbow hard feels like, or what it feels like after sitting on your hands for a few minutes. That feeling of your limb "going to sleep" has a similar kind of tingly sensation, but that doesn't last long and is fairly localized. My new sensations could last for an hour or longer, and could be happening with either hand, or both legs, simultaneously. And their intensity could increase, subside, and increase again. I was experiencing these strange feelings in my extremities, but the notion that MS had taken up permanent residency in my whole body had not registered yet. There were days when I felt fine with no symptoms at all, which lulled me into the fantasy that MS was not such a terrible thing to have, and that I could handle it without a problem.

I had seen firsthand so many individuals who were so much worse. I just could not believe that this was a big deal for me. I was sure I would be able to tolerate what ever was to come, because it was not going to be much at all.

"Janis, I'm not like them. I'm not going to get that bad. I'm not. I would be like them already if I was headed in that direction. The people we know who have MS got it when they were a lot younger than I am. There's nothing to worry about. I have a mild case. Simple as that." I tried to allay her concerns and mine. But, I wasn't so convincing with myself as things progressed.

37

I BEGAN FEELING a really bizarre sensation, like a strong electrical charge, that started at the back of my neck, and traveled the full length of my spine. It was different than anything I had ever felt in my life.

I've been shocked several times over the years – stringing Christmas lights, car battery terminals. This had resembling effects, but it was over and over, whenever I wanted it to happen. I could cause it by tucking my neck underneath my chin. I discovered this phenomenon soon after my diagnosis. It is called L'Hermittes Response. It does not hurt at all. It is quite painless, but it just feels weird. I was fascinated by its feeling and the way I could make it happen whenever I wanted to as long as I was vertical. I could lower my head and feel a jolting buzz, and no one on earth would have any idea that I was feeling something really strange. Not bad, not painful, just a very unusual electric-like sensation. I felt it sitting or standing. I would always feel it when I needed to go to the bathroom and urinate.

All of these new physical, never felt before in my life-type feelings were screaming "HELLO! THIS IS MS!! WAKE UP AND

SMELL THE COFFEE!!" The pain in my legs was increasing, the strength and length of time of tingles was increasing. Spasms in my legs at night kept me from sleeping for hours, or I would wake up with spasms and not be able to go back to sleep. Fatigue increased daily it seemed and I started the day tired and became feeling more tired as the day progressed. My gait became awkward with small, baby steps and poor balance. Somewhere along the way I realized my body was out of control, it was certainly out of MY control.

"You are a walking time bomb about to explode at any moment!" I believed my bomb had dropped. No doubt about it. Dr. Nunez was right after all.

Acceptance of my MS still came slowly, but it was so real there was no way to deny it. Not to anyone else, not to myself. As long as I could hide it from others, it wasn't so bad, and it was like I didn't have it, because I didn't look any differently than when I was normal. But, when the pain and fatigue in my legs made me look like I was limping badly all the time I had to open up with those around me. I had to explain to them what I had and how it affected me. I had to teach those around me about my MS. I had to explain my diagnosis, my prognosis and what I could do about it. I had to reassure them that I could still function. I just moved a little slower and more cautiously, I could not lift or carry as much. I had to accept and tell others what was going on with me.

With every person that I talked to about my disease it became easier. I began to be more willing to talk about it. I felt more comfortable. I relaxed. I did not need to hide the facts any longer. I had nothing to hide, really. It was silly to not talk about it.

I had been contacted six months earlier by a local reporter to give her a story about my MS, and I had declined. Now I was ready to talk to the press about how I was handling my MS. It was too obvious to try and continue to hide it, so why even try? I had finally reached the point of acceptance and had overcome my denial. It wasn't easy, and it didn't happen all at once. I'm not even sure when it happened, but I am glad I am now past it. I was now open and candid about my MS, and am perfectly willing to speak about it to anyone. It was a long arduous, punishing process that I had worked my way through.

Denial is not just a state of mind. It is also a period of time, a stage which has a beginning, a middle and an end, which may be precise or in little chunks falling away one at a time. Overcoming denial was not as easy as wiping words off a chalkboard. Acceptance came slowly. I thought I could whisk away what MS was to me, but that was not the case at all.

I had to go through a lot of questions, a lot of self analysis, anger, depression, doubt, research, education, resolve, courage, understanding and determination before I got to the point of acceptance and openness. There were many months following my diagnosis when I knew I had it, but I could not get the words out of my mouth to tell others. I could not define what I was feeling physically or psychologically. I knew no one would understand. No one else I knew ever felt like this. I was sure of that.

Making things even more difficult was that fact that my symptoms were changing frequently. My body was constantly talking to me in a foreign, unheard language. There were times I was in pain. Not usual, familiar pain. This is different pain. Searing pain. Weakening pain. Bring tears your eyes type pain. A totally new set of kinds of pains I've never felt before.

There were times I felt pins and needles under my skin in my arms or legs or feet. I had terrible headaches different than any I had ever had before. My legs would suddenly jump over and over involuntarily. My thighs would tighten up so stiff I could only take little short 10-12 inch steps, and I would have to sit down often and rest while walking.

I developed a great fear that when I walked somewhere I would not be able to walk back to where I started. But, I never knew how far I could go, so I worried whenever I went any where. I did not know my limits and my capabilities. I lived constantly in fear and doubt. Even though outwardly, I looked normal and quite healthy, inside of me I was living a nightmare.

The thought of death consumed me, not death per se. My death. I knew it was coming. I didn't know when or how long it would take, but I knew it was coming, and probably a lot sooner than I had been expecting.

I wrote several poems about my death. Snow Covered Mountains was the last one I wrote before I published my first book:

Snow Covered Mountains

I want to see snow covered mountains
And I want to see skies of blue.
I want to smell the salt of the ocean
And I want to spend time with you.

I've been told my time is short.
And I'll be passing on.
The things I love will still be here
But, soon I will be gone.

I thought I had a lot more time.

I made a lot of plans.
My candle's burning down too soon
I just don't understand.

I want to see snow covered mountains
And I want to see skies of blue.
I want to feel the sun on my face,
And I want to spend time with you.

I look at my life –I get flashes.
I see all the things that I've done.
Of all the people that mean something to me
You are the only one.

I want to see snow covered mountains
And I want to see skies of blue.
I want to dance just one more dance,
And I want to spend time with you.

I decided to take the family to The Magic Kingdom in Orlando, Florida. It was less than three hours drive from our home. We went there as often as we could, several times a year. One of my favorite parks is Epcot. I especially liked the American Pavilion in the World Showcase at the far end of the park in between Italy and Japan.

After eating a terrific meal at the China pavilion and watching the 360 degrees film of their country we went to see if the Voices of Liberty singers would be there, and they were just about ready top start. I don't know why, but as they start singing a capella, no accompaniment, and the world stopped. I started to cry. Big tears that I couldn't stop flowed down my face. The entire 15 minute performance I was pouring out tears like a faucet. I thought the music was beautiful. Their harmony was incredible. I'd never been a crier. Not like this. This was a new MS thing. It was a cry of joy, not sorrow. I didn't cry for me. I just heard such moving sounds, I was overwhelmed and mesmerized. I cried from appreciation and enjoyment. I was awestruck. I felt beautiful music in every square inch of my body. I could not stop or control my tears.

38

THE NEXT WEEK I decided to hit some golf balls on the driving range on my way home. Janis and the girls were off doing something and the weather was nice. For nearly 50 years, my practice tee habits hadn't changed since my early days hitting old balls at Coffeyville Country Club.

Plop, plop, plop.....The balls fell into the bucket after I'd paid my money. I carried my bag and the balls to the chipping green, and I started chipping short little 25 foot 7-iron chip shots toward the target pin. Then I pulled out my sand wedge and decided to hit a few flop shots.

Normally, I used the sand wedge on the range, not the practice green. For no reason, and without thought, I changed my usual practice plan and hit sand wedges. I was standing, facing the parking lot, but the cars were parked way over on the other side past the green.

Then two things, the worst of all possible things, happened simultaneously. From out of nowhere a family appeared and crossed the walk way in line with my shots. Not yet seeing them because my head was down, I skulled the ball, hitting it with the blade such that the ball flew straight with no trajectory just above the ground. In stead of hitting it 25 feet, I hit it about 40 yards. My ball hit a young girl, age 11, square in the forehead. I yelled, but it was too late.

"Oh, God, I'm sorry. Is she OK?" I ran toward them.

Both parents gave me a look of absolute horror. Rightfully, so.

The mother turned her daughter around away from me. The young girl with her hands over her face sobbed loudly. The father directed his attention at me.

"Let's go inside. You idiot. I want to make a report and turn you in."

I was shaking. I went along without saying anything. I felt horrible, but that wasn't going to help.

"This maniac hit my daughter. I want him arrested! Now!"

"What happened?" the pro asked once we were both inside.

The father took charge quickly." He hit my daughter. He was shooting at us. Call the police." Then he turned toward me. "You're too dangerous to be out there. You're a menace to society. They should lock you up. My daughter could have been killed!"

The head pro, cool and direct, talked to the enraged father. "Now let's calm down. You sit over there, he said talking to me, and I'll get to you later. I need to make a phone call and then I'll get your information." He indicated a chair for me, and I sat in it obligingly with no comment.

I at least knew enough not to enrage this guy any more than he already was. *Silence was the best approach. Don't give him anything to feed on. Don't stoke this guy's fire.* I wished the room had been twice as large. I needed to be as far from him as possible for my own safety.

A sheriff did come, but I was not arrested. There were no signs telling the public not to do what I did. There were no laws broken.

It was just a careless, foolish, totally avoidable accident. It was completely my fault.

The father gave him his information and he left. I spoke to him next. I was as apologetic as I could be. I told him I knew I was wrong, and it was my fault. I answered all his questions, and I asked him for the parents address and her name so I could send an apology letter. He acquiesced.

"I think you better not come around here for a while, ya hear? Wait till things settle down."

"Yes, sir. Thank you." I knew he was right about that, too. It was a total lack of good judgment on my part.

I wanted to give him an anology that it I had been shooting baskets in a gymnasium, and tried to make a lay-up, it would have been like I had thrown the basket ball so badly the ball flew into the highest row of bleachers, but I decided against it. I promised it would never happen again and I left.

I wrote the girl a letter, asking her for forgiveness, and I told her how sorry I was. I told her I had been hit four times and one of them caused a concussion. But, I had been playing for over 50 years and it was the greatest game in the world. I told her not to let my one terrible shot ruin her continuing to enjoy and to learn the game. I extolled the virtues of the golf and I hoped she got to read it. Might have been seized and discarded by the father without even opening it. That's something I'd never know.

The incident made me realize I was potentially dangerous, to myself and to others. My decision to shoot a ball in that direction was something I would have never done early in my life. My God. I've been teaching safety in my work for years. I gave over 2000 golf lessons when I was a pro without any accidents. I've never caused harm to another person intentionally or accidentally. I was the

Safety Director for my company. What was wrong with me??????
Why did I do that???? How could I unthinkingly change a strict
regimen of practicing, developed over time and never varying once
for some forty years? Why then? Why that day? More importantly,
how did I keep myself from making that kind of wrong move again?
Was this an example of the cognitive impairments referred to in the
MS side effects? I definitely believe it was. Very definitely.

I've never hurt anyone before. I've never hit another person with
an errant shot. I know better. I knew it and I thought I was skilled
enough to not hit anything that far off. I thought I was. Obviously,
no longer was this to be the case. Was my mind more affected
than I realized? Was MS more than just physical changes? Was I
affected in my decision making? How could I guard against that?
How would I know when I wasn't thinking right, when I was the
one doing the judging about my own thinking?

I never heard from her family. I was never sued. I could only
pray she had a complete recovery, and I hoped some day she would
go out to the golf course later on in her life and laugh about it as
no big deal.

Again, I did not make the connection that my lack of judgment
was an indication of an MS cognitive symptom gone awry. It would
only be much later, after much reading and contemplating and
making other bad decisions, did the invisible signs and the far
reaching affects of my disease begin to dawn on me. This was
another part of "the bomb" that Dr. Nunez had referred to.

Some time after my diagnosis had firmly set in and the realities
of its consequences were swimming in my mind, a profound sense
of urgency swept over me.

I shared my thoughts with Janis. "I should do what I can do
while I can still do it." I did not how long my window of opportunity

was. I did not know how long I would live. I did not know how long I would still be able to walk, or work, or run, or do anything that I could do at that time. I realized that there was no certainty to these questions, and no one on earth could answer them. But, I was not going to let MS steal from me those things that I wanted to do, but had not yet done.

To quote a phrase from Shakespeare's "Macbeth, " …If it' twere done when 'tis done, then 'twer well it 'twer done quickly." So, we began attending concerts, eating lavishly, making plans, jamming as much fun as possible into our lives. I began thinking of what I wanted to do in my life that was still unfinished, or still on my "things to do in my life" list.

Coincidentally, my son, Weslee, contacted me with one of those items. He must have been thinking the same things I was. His timing couldn't have been more perfect.

39

"DAD, REMEMBER HOW you always said you wanted to play golf in Scotland. I think we should start planning. What do you think?"

One of my dreams yet fulfilled was to play golf at St. Andrews, in Scotland. He knew that only too well, as we had talked about it many times over the years. I have a painting of St. Andrews in my office. It made sense.

"I love it, and I love you for suggesting it. Let's do it."

"OK. I really think it's a great idea. Let's get some options, times, places, costs." I knew he was serious. It was the right time. I couldn't put it off any longer. I thought it was something I would do when I retired, but my horizon has been compressed who knows how much. I'd better do it now, while I still can.

I had long since moved from the PGA to having an MBA, and had left the golf business behind me. But, the dream was still there. While I was a pro I studied the game. I was an expert at the rules. I educated myself with golf's history. I knew all the old famous players by name. Even though know he's dead, but I would recognize Walter Hagen if he walked in the door.

I had a reputation for being a very successful and effective teacher with men, women, children, and even disabled players. I was a student of the game and knew all the teaching methods and shots. I loved golf. I revered golf. I slept golf, I ate golf, I dreamed golf. Golf was my life. Still. I just didn't play as well or as often. It was only fitting, with all of this inside of me, that I would visit the home of golf.

When my son called and suggested we go to Scotland, I did not hesitate. Even though my game had fallen to where I could not break 80, I knew I had to go. We began planning in November, and had made firm plans by December to go to Scotland in April.

Scotland is where the game of golf was first created over 600 years ago. St. Andrews. The Royal and Ancient is the most famous golf course in the world. My dream was about to come a reality.

It was a long flight overnight and I watched the same movie three times, "Drumline" starring Nick Cannon. I couldn't sleep. Probably a combination of excitement and discomfort trying to sleep sitting up. But, it was a small sacrifice for the chance to get there.

Janis and the girls didn't come for a variety of reasons. This was a golfing trip. This was my dream come true. Golf is not their passion. There's not a great deal of family entertainment where we were going. War was imminent in Iraq and Janis didn't think we should be traveling anywhere right now. No. It was a special time for a father and his son. There would be other times for family fun.

We had to fly through Paris to get to Scotland, so we decided to enjoy some sightseeing and spent one day visiting the Louvre and Notre Dame. Mona Lisa looked exactly like the thousand or so pictures of her I'd already seen, but it was special seeing the original. It was an awfully long walk from the entrance to see her, and I walked up more stairs than I could count, but when I got that close, why not go all the way?

The Louvre was an enormous and impressive structure laid out in the shape of a horseshoe. We walked what seemed like many blocks, and climbed a mountain of stairs inside which culminated in getting to the end of the long corridor. I could have taken a half a day just peering at the enormous paintings on the walls that we passed by on our way to the final destination.

It seemed like more than just a museum. It was itself a part of history, and it contained thousands of pieces of history. If I was more prone to studying art, I could have stayed wandering slowly along there for days. I watched several artists copying paintings, exactly like what they were standing in front of. I wanted to talk to them, but I didn't. My legs were tiring and I could feel them swelling up.

I saw escalators too late as I had already made my way to Da Vinci's "heralded lady" and back nearly to the front entrance before I noticed them. That was OK. It gave me more time to take in all the view, one step at a time.

For April it was a warm day in Paris, perhaps 75 degrees and I started weakening after climbing many stairs and walking long corridors to see the most famous painting in the world. My steps shortened, my legs tightened up, my pace slowed and I could not walk more than a few hundred feet without having to stop and rest. Fortunately, I had brought a neat little folding cane that converted into a seat and I used it each time I needed to stop and rest.

"Hold up, Wes. Need a break here." My legs felt like telephone poles. I was walking with the grace and coordination of Frankenstein, except his legs were longer.

"OK, Dad, take it easy. No rush." He had been watching me. We traveled in chunks with many stops about 100-200 feet at a time, with 2-3 minutes of rest while I sat on in between.

After stumbling for many blocks and taking far too long to walk back to the hotel I was very concerned that I may not be able to have the strength to play golf. Maybe not even one hole. We cut out the part of trip walking to the Eiffel Tower. I gazed at it in the distance towering over the city while I was sitting on park bench. I wanted to get a better look at a nice grouping of local paintings displayed on a stretch of pavement overlooking the Seine, but time resting was more needed at that moment. Going to the Eiffel Tower was definitely out of the question.

Great, I worried! I had flown all that way, from Florida to Paris, and I may not have been able to get out on the course in Scotland. Pain and stiffness ran through my legs relentlessly. After further worry, I settled on being extremely positive about it. It was great just to be with my son for a week. It was going to be great just to be there, and if I couldn't play, so be it. At least I could see St. Andrews. I wasn't going to let myself be disappointed. Whatever happened would happen. C'est la Vie.

We had dinner at the Royal Madeleine Restaurant and Bistro recommended by the gentlemen who checked us in to our hotel. I had the best French onion soup of my life. What else would you expect in Paris?

To my unanticipated pleasure temperatures in Scotland were much cooler than in France, upper 40's and 50's, and my fatigue and leg cramps were gone. I was feeling stronger and my stride was normal for the rest of the trip. Even when I got tired, I sat on my portable chair and recovered in a few minutes.

We had plans for playing five different courses in six days, and doing some sight-seeing in Edinburgh in one middle day during the trip. In the next six days we would see Gulane, North Berick, Saint Andrews –the Old Course, Saint Andrews -The New Course and Carnoustie. There was also an amazing huge castle built over a thousand years ago at the highest point in Edinburgh. We absolutely had to see it.

"It's a wonderful walk passing all kinds of shops," a couple we met at the airport told us. "You'll find a delightful assortment of shops, pubs and restaurants on the Royal Mile as you walk down the hill from the castle. There are several stores with famous Scottish plaids and scarves. You'll listen to a man dressed in plaid kilts playing a bagpipe on a street corner. He's always there. Don't miss him. Go see the Scotch shop. It's got every kind of Scottish whiskey you can think of and a lot more."

I mentioned that I wondered if I'd see my Dad's favorite Scotch, Cutty Sark. Hadn't thought of it in years, but I could still see a vivid memory of the trash full of empty yellow and green bottles that I took outside out of our house and put it by the trash can.

"Yepper, sure enough. It's there among them, you'll find it."

"And do go all the way to the bottom. All the way to Hollyrood Palace where the Royal family stays several times each year. Beautiful castle it is. Now, it can't get any more Scottish than that, can it? Aye?"

"Thanks. We'll do it." We said good bye and walked off deciding we'd just heard some pretty interesting things worth seeing. We took their advice.

At the airport we picked up our transportation for the trip. "Wes, Can you drive a stick?"

"Nope."

"Wanna learn?"

"Nope."

"They didn't teach you that at Georgia Tech?"

"Nope."

"I guess I know what I'm going to be doing. Hop in."

Driving a small unfamiliar rental car with a stick shift, sitting on the right side of the car, gear shift in my left hand and whizzing down the left side of the road was a first. I did all the driving. Wes did all the navigating. This was a potentially very dangerous team of blind leading the blind. We were in for an adventure.

"OK. Dad. According to this map they gave us you will come to two round-a-bouts. Go through the first one and then take the second left after that." Moments later....... "Left. Left. Left," I said. "You missed it! Turn around. Watch out! OK. Again. Left. No, Left."

This turned out to be an interesting challenge in itself that we weren't expecting. Wes didn't realize how weak my legs were. Pumping the shift and break with my left leg, while accelerating with my right foot became hard to do, and took all my concentration. I had not driven a stick shift in many years. And, thanks to British mentality, I was sitting in the right seat of the car, shifting gears with my left hand while steering with the right. Everything was backwards.

Turning, steering and listening to his directions, seeing traffic signs that were unfamiliar while catching a few sights of the beautiful country along the way simultaneously was occasionally more than my not-so-good-at-multitasking brain could handle.

This was another invisible sign of MS. My cognitive abilities were compromised, but there was no way to recognize them at this early juncture. As with so many other symptoms, it was still premature for me to put all the threads together to see the big picture which explained so many things that had made no sense before.

Somehow, Wes and I got everywhere we were going safely. Fairly safely. Once I hit a hedge pretty hard. I ran over a bunch of curbs. Nearly hit a few cars. I scared Wes to death a few times. And, I'm quite sure I disturbed an otherwise calm day for numerous drivers behind me, who were quick to honk at me when I slowed to wait and process Wes's instructions. I was advancing further onto unfamiliar narrow roads, confusing traffic signs, a meshwork of round-a-bouts and small villages with parked cars and buildings protruding very close to me as we whizzed by them. With the grace of God watching over us, we were unharmed.

I couldn't find the reverse. I guessed these new cars weren't made like the old ones I drove 30 some years ago. Perhaps it came in a diabolical or convoluted way that was designed to intentionally confound us foreigners. Reverse or "R" was nowhere to be seen. I couldn't just pull down or towards me and go backwards. So, for the first two days we parked on inclines where there was space behind me, or in front of me, so I could put it into neutral and get it started by using gravity.

I finally asked a stranger walking by where the reverse was in our car. He showed me in two seconds how you grab the stick and pull straight up. He was very friendly. I'm sure he thought we were just a couple of stupid Americans. Maybe we were.

We had caddies each day except the one day that we had an electric golf cart. I skipped playing two holes two of the days to rest while my son played up and back and rejoined me to complete the round. I did walk as much as I possibly could, and was proud that my body did not give out on me once.

I was not playing great golf. I wasn't expecting to. I hit a few good shots here and there. I hit a lot of good drives. I showed I could still hit the driver 250-275 yards depending on the wind. Far more importantly, I WAS THERE. In Scotland. Playing St. Andrews, the Old Course, the New Course, Carnoustie, and more. I was living my dream. A dream that I had for nearly 50 years was coming true. I played courses where many great players had been. It was a almost surreal being there.

I walked across the stone Swilcan Bridge on the 18th hole at St. Andrews where every championship player passed. We stopped there for s moment and my caddie took pictures of Wes and I on the bridge and again on the 18th green with the Royal and Ancient's club house in the background. The next year Jack Nicklaus would stand on that same bridge while playing the British Open and wave farewell as he planned to soon retire.

No one could ever take that away from me. It was a dream fulfilled. A trip full of memories, stories and gratifications I will never regret. A trip that I am forever grateful to my son for joining me and helping to make it happen. MS be damned, I was living my life and my dreams.

Truth be known, spending a week with Wes, my son, just the two us, was something that, well, we could have enjoyed if it had rained every day. We can always have a good time and make the best of it.

And, it was just in time, although we did not know it then how propitious it turned out to be. One year later my physical abilities deteriorated to the extent that I could not have made that trip again. I can still swing a club, but it's not likely that I could walk one hole without falling, and likely could not have had the strength to play even nine, let alone eighteen holes walking with a caddie. If

I had put off the trip until the following year, I would never have even attempted to go.

It is very unlikely that I will ever return to Scotland. Both my age and the progressive nature of my disease are working against me. Barring a miraculous recovery I would never be able to play there, as they frown on slow players, and at my speed of walking I would be courteously asked to pick up my ball and go home, for good. Electric carts are rare, and I was lucky the day I did get one. But, now that doesn't matter one scintilla. I did it! I did it once and that is enough for me to last a lifetime.

The main thing is I set a goal and made it happen. I did something very special for myself. Despite the risks, it was worth it. My MS did not take away living my dream, my good time or my joy. I'll treasure the memories the rest of my life and be proud about it.

40

RETURNING TO THE New York airport, I had to go through customs and go through my golf bag and my suitcases with the security guards. I had to do basically the same thing in Atlanta a few hours later. But, I had to stand in two separate lines – one for the golf bag and another line for the suitcase. This became a slow, tedious and tiring exercise.

My legs hurt. They burned constantly. It helped a little to sit on my cane, but in a few minutes I had to get up and move positions several feet down from where I just was. Got up and shifted down the line, down, up and down again. It hurt either way I did it.

I was sitting on my folding cane/chair for about 30 seconds. Then I stood up, pushed my suitcase, walked four feet, and sat down again. I plodded about 200 feet through step one, getting my suitcase inspected. My legs were painfully hurting, searing, burning. Rising up and down puts more stress on them. There was no way to escape the pain I was feeling.

Then they told me I had to check in the golf bag at a different location, on a different floor. My flight was getting close to boarding.

I was getting anxious. When I got on the next floor I ask for directions. Things start getting hairy.

"Here's my ticket. Here's my golf bag. I'm about to miss my plane. Can you help me?"

A lady at the customer service desk quickly realized the urgency of my situation.

"Oh, and I'm handicapped. Can you help me with that, too?" She gave me a stub for the bag. She never questioned why a handicapped person would be carrying a golf bag.

She spoke to someone on a walkie-talkie. "I need a wheel chair NOW." It came quickly. She pushed me for about a hundreds yards nearly running full pace and a young man pushed me the rest of the way, following her orders to get me to the gate, pronto. We arrived to an empty gate area. I entered the plane's door holding out my ticket.

"Go ahead. Get in." My ticket was snatched up. The door was closed and latched immediately behind me. "Come this way, right over here." I was shown a seat, and the plane began its approach down the runway. Every second counted. I just made it thanks to some wonderfully helpful people.

41

"HI, EVERYONE. I'M home!"

Janis and the kids hugged me as I walked in the door. It was great to be home, but the magic was over. Back to the usual routine. Back to reality. Back to responsibilities. Back to dealing with my MS. It was worth every bit of it to go.

I began attending monthly MS support group meetings offered by several local groups. They were scheduled for early evening and I could make them if I got out of work by 5 PM.

I've always been conscientious about being on time for meetings. I've always been a punctual person. Mom made me that way, in reverse. She made me late for everything and I couldn't stand it. Now I try every way I can to avoid the embarrassment I suffered as a child. Being on time is a high priority with me, even when it's not really that important to any one else.

It was nearing 5 pm at work on the Wednesday of one of the MS meetings and I met an unexpected stumbling block. Allison, an accountant, had decided to stay late and work beyond her usual 5 o'clock leaving. This posed a problem to me, because I couldn't lock up and set the alarm until she left. If she stayed I'd miss my meeting.

"Allison? What are you doing?

"Working late."

"What do you mean? You can't stay! You must go. You didn't ask to stay late and I have a meeting to make. I have to get out of here, like now!"

"Well, I have to get my work done. I'm a little behind, you know."

"I don't care. I'll talk to your supervisor tomorrow. You must go. Now! Come on, move it."

She didn't budge.

"You can't just sit there. It's time to leave. You have no right to stay without prior notice to me. You will screw up my evening, I have made arrangements. I have checked with a lot of other people to be able to leave at this time. With everyone but you, it seems. You must go."

I was vociferous. I was loud and demanding. I was shaking. I pressed harder and got more personal. "It's very unprofessional for you to do this. No communication. You can't go around assuming you can do whatever you want. I mean, really."

"What's wrong with you, Mr. Knapp? I've never seen you like this? You are not yourself."

"I don't know what you mean. Just please go. OK?"

She left begrudgingly. I wrote a scathing letter to her supervisor the next day. The issue never came up again. I made it to the MS meeting a few minutes late, but, I didn't miss anything.

I had entered into a new phase of my life where too many things were happening at once and I couldn't handle it. But, I didn't realize how much I was reacting to it in ways that were not normal for me.

My walking deteriorated more. My stride was choppy in the morning and as the day marched forward my steps became shorter and shorter. Janis bought a used wheel chair for me. I wasn't in favor of it, but it felt good to ride and not be put in a position where I was in constant pain. Walking was now always painful. Standing was excruciating. It was just a question of how much could I endure.

She pushed me or one of my daughters would push me, or they would take turns. Anywhere outside of the house when we were together, excluding work, I was riding in a wheel chair. I was in a Catch 22. I hated it and I didn't think I needed it, but it sure felt good. I couldn't walk very far or get anywhere quickly without it.

People looked at me differently. Actually, they didn't usually look at all. They looked away and avoided eye contact. I was lower to the ground than all but the littlest of toddlers, so my eyes were lower than all the other people I was around. I didn't like that. I couldn't see past the person in front of me.

My unyielding attitude didn't just hold true for Allison, I was becoming more and more intolerant with everyone, especially my wife.

"Why don't you step back and see the big picture, Steve. You've changed. You are not the person I fell in love with and married. You've changed a lot more than you realize. Can't you see it?"

This has been building up for months. I had no idea how my MS had changed me so much, but I was in complete denial about it.

"No. You've changed. You can't keep the house up. It's not even safe for me to walk around. I don't like how you handle our money. I don't like how you discipline the kids. I mean, I can't agree with anything you do anymore. I want a divorce. I've decided to contact an attorney who would see I'm right and help me get out of this relationship."

She didn't deserve any of that but I couldn't see what was real and what wasn't. Janis and I argued constantly. I knew it was all her fault and I filed for divorce. She was the cause of my black and blue toes. She was why I didn't have enough money. I couldn't sleep because she was keeping me up. I was yelling at her and she couldn't see why.

It wasn't about fidelity. We were both loyal to each other. It was about compatibility. She was driving me crazy. Everything she did made no sense. I wasn't going to live the rest of my life under the kind of duress I was under. It was all her fault. She'd lost her mind. Or, so I thought at the time.

After a few months, strangely, she changed. She was polite to me. We agreed on things. We were respectful and loving to each other, like before. I couldn't divorce her then. This was my old wife back again. I stopped the divorce and pledged that I would never do that again. I couldn't go through with it. We were back being friends and lovers again. Fortunately, I came to my senses. I wasn't able to see how I had changed. This was another invisible cognitive element that had silently slipped into my new MS life.

42

I WAS ALSO trying to publish a poetry book in my spare time that I had been working on for four years. Its title was "Good Poetry That Makes Sense." It was a compilation of 100 of my best poems. The timing was terrible. I had it placed on Amazon.com and Barnes and Noble.com and that's as far as I got. I had no interest or energy to get it off the ground. It did not sell well because nobody knew about it. I didn't promote it at all.

Work offered its usual pressures and I floated from project to project and varied responsibilities not really taking much initiative. I could not evaluate myself realistically. I couldn't see myself. I didn't know who I was anymore. I could discern I was not the usual me, physically or psychologically, but doing the right thing to change for the better was beyond my capability.

There were several more outbreaks at home and Janis wife recognized my sudden changed personality on several occasions. We brought this up with Dr. Nunez.

"He's like living with Dr. Jeckle and Mr. Hyde. I never know what to expect. I don't know him any more." Janis was being truthful to Dr. Nunez.

She suggested I take Wellbutrin. It's a drug for depression, and she said it would take the "highs" and "lows" out of my day. After I started taking it I became more stable, more rational and in better control of myself. It didn't cure all my problems, but it made a huge difference in my behavior. Cognitive issues were still impossible for me to recognize at the onset, but I was increasing my awareness of my instablilty.

I didn't realize how different I became, but I must have been a real bear to be with. I found myself losing my temper with less self control for months before I started taking the prescription. It didn't take much to set me off. That's not me. I'm usually Mr. Cool -as – a - Cucumber. One of the traits Janis liked about me was how calmly I handled high pressure situations. What happened?

After about a month we realized the Wellbutrin wore off about 5 PM, and the doctor recommended taking one at 7 AM and a second dose at 5 PM. That even worked better because I had become aggressive and hard to deal with when I arrived home in the evenings. Taking two doses a day, one in the morning and one in the evening did the trick.

I was showing two distinctly different personalities - one with the Wellbutrin and the other one without it. I could be manic one minute and depressive the next. I could be calm and quiet and suddenly explode. I still couldn't tell the difference in me. Janis and the kids could spot it in seconds. It's happened enough times I believed them. When they told me it's time to take a pill, I didn't argue. I just reached for the Wellbutrin bottle.

Returning home in Florida after the Scotland trip meant being subjected to higher temperatures, even much higher than I had felt in Paris. Florida weather was turning to summer-like conditions with temperatures over 90 degrees and very high humidity. And, with the heat came a plethora of completely new sensations, and the ones I had been feeling were much stronger. I gave them names because they reminded me of the 4th of July.

I was pretending I had purchased an assorted pack of special fireworks. They were unique because they'd go off on the inside, imploding in my legs, my hands, my arms, my thighs. There are no colors, no noises, no smoke or fire - only sensations. I opened them up and set them off, one at a time. The Snakes were always interesting. They started at a point in my body and slowly moved up with a lot of consternation and eruption without going very far. For me these were electrical surges that occurred usually in my lower legs and calves. Once in a while the Snakes visited my arms, too. They seem to start with a lot of determination, but ended shortly and without notice.

Lady Fingers were mild little pops that struck me most anywhere in my legs and arms. They were not strong, and once in a while, they fizzled and nothing happened. They were sudden bursts of electrical spasms, always unexpected, but never very harsh. They did cause embarrassing, clumsy moments when drinking a cup of coffee, or opening a door.

The Roman Candles offered another category of 4th of July surprises. Starting at the hip, or thigh, left or right, they went streaming down the leg in an increasing surge and burst close to the ankle or foot. There was enough stimulation to make my foot jump, sometimes, or just hang suspended until the feeling passed. They followed in turn by another and then another, and could continue and last for quite a long time. I felt these Roman Candles most when sitting or just before going to sleep.

Finally, there were the Sparklers. These amazing wands were able to make thousands of points of light all feel tingly sensations at the same time.

The Sparklers could increase or decrease in their intensity, they could speed up or slow down in their occurrence, and they could shift and move from one part of a body to another. I felt Sparklers from my toes to my fingertips, and almost anywhere in between. Sometimes they radiated heat, like a blow torch, and sometimes they are as cool as ice. I could have many Sparklers active at one time. They were unpredictable.

I had good days and bad days, but the fireworks were always there, lying inside of me, waiting for an unknown spark to set them off. They may be at rest for a while, but they would always awaken and come back. They were at times very confusing. They were at times a distraction and an annoyance. I made one choice about the fireworks that was consoling to me. It was far better, I believe, to feel the effects of them – the Snakes, the Lady Fingers, the Roman Candles and the Sparklers, than it would be to have no feelings at all. Most doctors agree that when the feelings are absent completely then the nerves are dead and, at that point, there is no chance of recovery. So, I'll accept these strange sensations and not complain. For the most part, however, it will be a show that no one but me will see, as all these crazy feelings are all inside of me and invisible to the world of the unknowing.

43

AS THE TEMPERATURE rose I was starting to react more to my body getting warmer and my sensations of "tingliness" in my legs, feet, toes, arms, hands, and fingers were getting stronger. On a scale of 1 to 10, I was feeling them at levels of 7 or 8, which, to me, was pretty strong. Sometimes they would come and go, and other times they would stay for an hour or more. When I lifted something heavy, I would feel sensations stronger than usual in my hands and arms.

When I mowed the lawn I would have sensations after coming inside. If I used the hedge trimmer, or the electric edger, or the weed eater, I would not feel anything unusual at the time, but as soon as I finished, the tingly feelings were especially strong. Like a 9. My arms and hands buzzed like the machine was still running in my hands, even though I had put it down and disconnected the power. At that level, I couldn't do much. It was impossible to ignore how strong the feelings were. They were a distraction at a 5 level, but at a 9 they were an unbelievable phenomenon. I just sat there and waited for the feelings to subside. I was in a spell, suspended in time, totally focused on what I was feeling. It was like having the Northern Lights displaying inside of me. No one could see anything different about me, but I was so alive with electricity, it is difficult to describe.

Janis and I attended a performance at Florida Atlantic University. It was the Boca Pops. We enjoyed listening to a variety of beautiful music played by a very talented orchestra. Every so often they would stop and we would clap. After three or four claps my hands would tingle so strongly I had to stop clapping. It took several minutes for the feelings to subside. Finally, I stopped clapping altogether and just listened. On one or two of the songs they played so loudly the noise pierced my ears and I had to cover my ears with my hands. It was embarrassing to my family who did not understand, but I was in great pain from the beautiful, but loud, music.

A few days later at the Town Center Mall in Boca Raton, Florida a few miles from where we lived I went shopping with my family. They were intent on looking for girls clothing which was not very exciting to me, so I sat down at a fountain where the corridor bends. A lady and her son threw some coins into the water.

Thoughts of my MS turned to coins lying in the waters of the fountain, cast by others hoping to make a wish come true. I started writing down all the thoughts that came to me and later I organized them.

The Eternal Mystique of Fountains and Coins

What is the illusive connection here? Where is the source of this ostensibly capricious power? And most importantly of all, what are the rules that define which and how a wish becomes reality? As I pass by a fountain in a well-traveled mall I ponder many things. Every coin is inextricably attached to a certain person's wish. How many wants, or whims, or needs, or desires, lie there in the flowing waters? How many lives are fated by the fountains and the coins? How many of these heartfelt wishes really do come true? How does it work– this wishing experience? Where do the secrets lie?

Does a nickel bring five times the wishes of a penny tossed into the fountain? Or can it be fives times as likely to make the wish come true? Does a dime's wish have more strength than a nickel's wish today? Does a quarter's wish rule over all, or will a penny do as well? Should you have to close your eyes real tight, or give a coin a kiss? What are the answers here within? Can the fountains hear your thoughts?

How long do wishes really last, before you know they can't come true? When does a wish lose all its hope? When is despair the only road? Do two coins have twice more power than one all by itself? Should you throw them both together? Will a wish have any chance to be if you tell it to another? Is it better to speak aloud, or keep it in your mind? Could an old wish just be standing in a queue, waiting for a better time for its fruition?

Or is it merely chance and luck that brings us what we hope for? Maybe the man in the black watch plaid is just wearing his lucky socks. Perhaps that lady with the sultry gait holds a lucky coin that bodes to her good fortune. Are coins and wishes simply daft superstitions, and fountains nothing more than elegant traps?

Although there is no apparent science or system to this scheme, fortune finds its way to certain souls whose wishes do come true. Dreams are launched on splashing coins, hopes make way secure. I stand before a magic fountain gazing at its awe. I have a pocketful of change and I have a very important wish to make. Would somebody, please, unveil its secrets and share with me the rules?

44

SLOWLY, I WAS coming to accept these feelings as something that accompanied my MS, and was just going to have to accept them. Then one day I noticed that the sun seemed to cover my arms with an invisible layer of heat. My arms were burning, although there was no apparent source of heat other than the sun, which I have been in all my life without this kind of sensation. I went inside and sat down. I felt the usual tinglies, and then the started to itch as if I had poison ivy on my arms. It would itch very strong for a few seconds, then when I scratched it, the itch would be cease, and the scratching felt good. But, then in a few seconds the itching would return a little stronger. So, after a few scratchings I knew I had to just bear it and hope it went away. But, curiously, the itches started happening all over my arms, legs, stomach, neck, hands, fingers, and shoulders. Basically, all over my body. No area was spared from this extreme itch.

I knew better than to touch, or rub, or scratch an itch My bout long ago with poison ivy taught me that lesson, but I was itching all over. It grew in its intensity and strength, and soon became so bothersome, and unbearable, that I had to scratch once in a while because it was too much to take.

There was nothing to see, no sores no rash, nothing on my skin. This itching went on all evening without any interruptions. I was trapped by my own itch. I went to bed itching like crazy. I could not sleep. There was no comfortable position to lie in, and I tossed and tossed for hours. I fell asleep from pure exhaustion about 4 am. The itch was finally gone.

I went through the next day feeling tired, and other than the usual tingly sensations, I had no other feelings until I got home. Around 7 pm, the itch returned. I had not been outside and was not exposed to the sun like yesterday, but the feelings were the same. I had to do something. The feelings were all internal, not topical. My wife tried blue ice, a muscle relaxant, to see if that helped, but it did not. I itched just as bad that night as the one before, and again could not go to sleep. It was unmerciful. If I scratched it, it felt good, then it itched worse. If I did not scratch it, it continued relentlessly, until I gave in and rubbed it. One of the worst areas of the itching was my palms. I couldn't stand it. The feelings were so strong it is hard to convey how intense the itching was. It became unbearable, at times, and I would find something rough, and rub my hands over the rough surface to ease, only momentarily, the itching. If I rubbed real hard, it might stop for a while, but would occur in some other area of my body. There was never complete relief. And, I was becoming dangerous to myself. I would scratch myself so hard there were real scratches showing on my arms.

I became a masochist. Day after day, I was fine until the evening, and then it would hit me so hard I had no recourse but to give in and scratch myself over and over every few moments when it was unbearable. Before the sun dipped in the evening, my ability to withstand the itching was challenged and I failed every time. Even my poison ivy that I caught years ago in Michigan was nothing compared to this.

After the sixth day in a row, I tried something novel. I was by the swimming pool, and the water was still pretty cool, so I dipped my arms deep into the water. I could not feel any itching. It was not comfortable lying on the edge of the pool with my arms in the water up to my arm pits, but there was a gracious reward that I had found a way to find some relief and comfort. From that idea I put five gallons of water in a bucket, put ice in it, and sat in the family room with my arms buried in the bucket. It worked! The secret was to keep my arms very, very cold. They did not itch when I withdrew my arms, so I dried them off. But, in about 15 minutes the itch returned to my arms. If I could focus on keeping my arms from not itching, the rest of my body did not itch, either. Maybe it was because I was keeping all of me cooler. I mentioned it to my neurologist, but he had never heard of this itching symptom before.

I remembered reading that heat was not friendly to MS, so maybe I was overheating each evening. I went to bed after several arm "dippings," and went to sleep for about 2 hours before waking up to itching arms. I went down stairs and plunged my arms again into the bucket of ice cold water for 15 minutes. Then I went back to bed. Fifteen minutes in the middle of the night bought me enough time to get enough sleep to make it until the next morning. It was the best solution I could think of.

Fortunately, the itching stopped after two weeks. One evening I came home and there was no itch. None. It has not returned again since it stopped. I know where to find my bucket fast if I ever needed it again. Hopefully, I won't. Since it mysteriously faded away I have heard of several MS folks who have had similar kinds of itches, and appreciated my sharing my solutions to them.

One of the feelings that kept changing throughout the day was my stamina. My varying degrees of strength and stamina puzzled me. I decided to look at this phenomenon as if they were in a bowl. The metaphor works to explain my energy to others. When the bowl was full I felt good, energetic, and normal. As I progressed through the morning the bowl began to empty. The more I walked, or lifted, or stood, the bowl would gradually become less full. Sitting and resting for a short time would refill the bowl, somewhat, but not to its original morning level. Still, it was an improvement. As the day moved forward into the late afternoon the bowl lost more and more of its volume. Little by little, small exertions would lower the level in the bowl. Large exertions, heavy exercise coupled with little rest would drain the bowl much sooner.

I never let the bowl become completely empty. Then I couldn't move at all. So, there was always a little reserve in the bottom of the bowl. But, some days if I let the bowl get too close to being completely empty, it did not refill all the way overnight. Then I started the next day with the bowl partly empty. That made that day a bit more difficult because I was at my best when the bowl was full. I didn't enjoy starting the day with my bowl only half-full.

I had to be careful not to let my bowl get too empty. It seemed to empty faster than it refilled. Only long periods of rest, or sleep, and minimal activity would allow the bowl to replenish itself. I felt so much better when my bowl was full. I wished I could keep my bowl full all the time. It seemed that the nature of my MS was to diminish the energy in my bowl. Proper foods, medications, ergonomics, vitamins, and less movement all helped, but nothing promised to keep my bowl full at all times.

I think my bowl has gotten a lot smaller since my MS has tried to take charge of my body. I always used to have a less than full bowl by the end of the day, but my bowl was never as empty as it is now. My bowl always refilled completely with a little rest. Now, I have to rest for much longer periods of time. And, my bowl used to not empty so fast. Sometimes I feel my bowl being nearly empty and it is only morning and I somehow have to keep it from being exhausted for the rest of the day. That never used to happen before. I used to store a lot more reserves in my bowl.

I was always judging what was left in my bowl. I questioned and doubted and tested my reserves. I didn't know where the bottom is. But, I felt its relative level. I felt its unscientific presence. It was inescapable. My bowl was always with me. I wondered how far I could go, and make it back. I worry about that a lot. I had to be on guard to know when to stop just before I fall. I had to evaluate my bowl in terms of my capabilities regularly. My limitations had changed, but they are still undefined. My bowl made that determination on an hour – by - hour basis.

No one can see my bowl, not even me. But, its effects are very visible. I got slower in my walk, I got tired more easily. It showed in my face, in my expressions, in my capabilities, in my strength, in my balance, in my confidence, in my coordination, in my stamina, in my temperament, in my self control. It has remolded me. My MS has changed my bowl, and my bowl has changed my life.

I cannot pinpoint the time or day this phenomenon began, but once it started, it had launched me into a continuum of time that has no beginning, and has no end. I was not coping well with my Multiple Sclerosis. I have been taking medication for 5 months. I was 53 years old at that time but I felt like I was 100 sometimes.

"Dad. Dad. Dad let's go out and play soccer in the yard." My daughters, Alexandria and Janna, pulled me out the front door.

"I'm sorry, I can't move. I've got to go back inside. I ache, I'm exhausted, I've got to go back inside and sit down. I can't handle being in this heat."

Their faces said it all.

"OK, Dad."

I used to love life, but the life I now live is not the life I used to love. It hurt that I couldn't go out and play with my kids. But, the reality is that I couldn't. Not only did I not feel like it, but I just didn't have the strength, the balance, the energy that I used to take for granted.

When I get out of bed in the morning I was stiff and tired and did not remember sleeping very much. It was as if I took a short nap, a light sleep and not very deep or hard. I wondered if I really did sleep, or was it so short I missed it completely. I crawled out of bed feeling like I want to go back in and get some real sleep, but I pushed that idea aside and shuffled out of the bedroom, holding the wall when needed, for balance. I showered, shaved, took my vitamins and got dressed. It's the same routine I have practiced for many years, but I now moved much slower, and more deliberate. I had to watch for things I could fall over, knock over, spill, or forget to do, so each action became an event which has to be thought out like I am doing it for the first time.

I drove to work and began the morning feeling exhausted from the get-go. I knew that as tired as I felt at that moment, it was the best I would feel all day. Every day started at a low base line, and went downhill from there. By noon I was so tired I had to sit and rest, even though I may had been sitting most of the morning anyway. I ate lunch and it gave me no extra energy, no lift. I no longer ate the delicious foods that I used to eat, because I now have to eat a strict diet, and most of it is rather bland. I have put myself on a healthy diet voluntarily, which will not give me headaches or make me ache later, but it was not the fun experience that it used to be for me.

I no longer eat cheeseburgers, steak, bacon or any red meat. I pass on chocolate chip cookies, pecan pie, ice cream and whipped cream. I don't eat French Fries, onion rings or other fried foods. I don't stop at KCF, I don't eat pizza, I don't drink any kind of soda pop, or beer, or liquor or wine. These foods and drinks will elicit a migraine within hours. It's not worth a few minutes of joyous taste for hours of pain.

Usually someone at work will catch me to talk and I have to oblige them by standing and listening.

Greg said,"Hey, Steve. Did you see the Marlins last night. Three home runs in one game. Did you see how far Mike Lowell hit that one in the 7th inning? Man, he doesn't look like he can hit one that far. He's not that big. We pounded them. You know it?"

"Yeah, we did." I couldn't even pretend to share his level of enthusiasm. I just nodded.

The pain increased with each minute of standing still. I was listening on the outside but wailing and wincing on the inside. I gracefully stepped away, get my activities handled and found my seat as soon as I could.

As the afternoon began my legs increased their very tingly sensations, my thighs were weak, and it was a bit difficult to stay focused, but I tried. Finally, it was time to go home and I was happy to sit in the car and take the weight off my legs as I drove on the interstate toward joining my family for the evening.

At home the day became a blur, and much of it passed by as if I were an observer, and not a participant. I don't feel the closeness and degree of control that was there before. When I was at home, I sat on the couch for most of the evening. My family and I interacted verbally, but my part in the activities of the house was relatively passive. I was so weak and fatigued I could only sit and watch. My family has been very good to me and I have come to appreciate their help, but I am saddened by my change of roles.

Whereas before my MS I was involved in many things that happened in the house, because I was the man, the strong guy, Mr. Fix It, Mr. Helpful, and Daddy – the guy who taught sports, swimming, playing catch, etc. I took out the trash, I cut down thick branches in the yard, I got on the roof, I climbed the ladder and changed out lights, I pressure washed the patio, and I put the chemicals in the pool. I had planned to play tennis and golf and basket ball with my daughters when they got a little older. I was the guy who stood on the ladder and put up the Christmas tree lights.

Now, my role had changed, my abilities had changed, as well. I had become Mr. Sit-On-The-Couch and Watch the TV. I was Mr. Couch Potato. I could help with homework, but I was very limited on the household chores. Outdoor physical exercise and other rigorous activities were not in the picture anymore, and were becoming less and less as time went on.

The evening waned and it was time for bed. I would go to the bedroom but it was becoming harder and harder to get undressed. The pants didn't come off easily any more because I couldn't lift my legs high enough. I nearly fell, often, trying to stand on one foot, fighting with a pant leg. It hurt my legs to stand and brush my teeth.

I collapsed into bed. I kissed my wife goodnight. I had no amorous inclinations. I was just too exhausted. I lay there but I soon I would have to get up to go to the bathroom. I noticed the clock and remembered its time. I slept somehow, but I soon awoke again. My legs were feeling jumping with spasms and they wake me up. A half hour passed. I lay in bed enduring the spasms, feeling my leg jump up every 20 -30 seconds like I had just been electrically shocked. I was thinking about work, and what needed to be done at home that I could do. An hour passed.

I had to get up and go to the bathroom again. I returned to bed and slept for a while. I awoke from a dream and looked at the clock. Twenty minutes has passed since I last looked at. I tried to remember the dream I just had. Something about when I was younger, and I was with friends I used to spend time with. I went back to sleep, but I don't sleep long. I got up because the air conditioner was too low and I was too cold. It was 4 am. I wondered how many minutes I had slept so far that night. It seemed like the night was very long. I used to wake up refreshed, with the feeling that I had slept for a short time, but eight hours had somehow quickly passed. I had slept so deeply I did not notice the time passing. Now, I noticed how shallow my sleep has become, and it felt like forever to get through one night. The night became an extension of the day, and I was just in a different place.

Finally, it was 5:30 am and I laid in bed wondering how a night could last so long. It was funny, but when I used to sleep all night long, it made a definitive cut-off between the night, and the beginning of the next day. The night and the day were different. Days were 24 hours. A day was split so that some of it was waking time, and some of it was sleeping time. Monday was different than Tuesday. Now, the night ran into the day, the day ran into the next night, and there was no cut-off. It was like one continuous day. Never ending. Never changing. I no longer lived a 24 hour cycle, I lived a day that had been continuously having its days and nights run together for many months. There was no Tuesday or Wednesday. It was all part of one long nondescript existence with no beginning and no end. I wanted to sleep for a long time and wake up feeling rested, but I felt just as tired when I got up as when I went to bed. What was the point? When did it end? When would that day ever end? Or did it keep going and going and going? I was trapped inside the seemingly eternal everlasting day, and I didn't know how to get out.

45

I TOOK A step back and started thinking about what had been happening to me. I was all alone going through all these horrible things. No one I knew was going through all that had been happening to me. I had become very depressed and didn't know it. I started writing about what I felt. I thought maybe I would understand it better. I thought maybe if I told others what I was going through, they might understand. I came to realize that this was no easy task.

I'd never given much thought to expressing how I felt. Now I was going to try to describe things that were new and different and no one I knew had a clue what I had, how I felt, what I had to face daily.

I put the following piece down on paper and decided it was a start. It described many thoughts in general terms that had become part of the MS life I was living.

NOBODY KNOWS

It is another day. I wake up feeling weak and tired. My legs are tingly and numb. I slowly get myself prepared for another arduous day. It requires much effort to take a shower and get myself dressed. Getting my slacks on and lifting my legs high enough to get them on becomes a challenge. It takes all the courage I can muster to put a smile on my face and walk into work trying to look like I'm ready to go. I start the day short on stamina, depressed in confidence, wondering if I can produce a full day's work. And fearful that I might fall, or make a mistake, or do something outrageously dumb. I have to write everything down and think through things very carefully. I am always on guard. I am a full-time actor.

And, no one knows it but me.

I walk from the car to the office and my feet shuffle a bit. I carefully lift my leg over the curb, knowing I have caught my foot on it before and fell, but no one was watching. By lunch time I am very tired and need to sit quietly and rest. I smile and carry a conversation while I eat, but my mind wanders, wonders and worries about how the rest of the day will go. I have to lift a light box of paper, and I do so easily, but cautiously, trying to be smooth and look coordinated. I used to be more coordinated without trying to appear so. Now that I have MS I have to be conscious and careful and deliberate with every movement, and I am. I can appear very clumsy and pitifully slow if I am not careful. I push myself to minimize the difference.

And, nobody knows it but me.

I am plagued by progressive fatigue each and every day. No matter what my level of energy is at the beginning of the day, it languishes. It is always less in the afternoon than in the morning, and less in the evening than in the afternoon. It is lost in spurts sometimes, when extra effort is required. It rushes out of me like a balloon losing its air.

My gait becomes choppy, and my stride becomes shorter. Concerned people think I have hurt my foot or my leg and ask what happened. I smile and make a quick passing excuse. It would take a long time to tell the truth, and I'm usually in a rush. In the evenings I sit and move as little as possible until it is time to go to bed. I am painfully exhausted.

And, nobody knows it but me.

I am ever conscious of my body. It talks to me sending me strange signals that I do not understand. I feel electrical current in my legs. I feel stiffness in my thighs. I get headaches of all kinds and from many different locations in my brain. I feel shooting impulses surging down from my thighs to my feet. My feet jump from the shock. Some part of my body is always sending me messages. At times they are mild and I try to be oblivious to them. When they are strong, I cannot block them out. They are involuntary and uncontrollable. Even when I sleep I am awakened to feel them talking to me. They have become inescapable reminders that I have MS. And thus, having MS is always in my consciousness. I am continually introspective about it.

And, no one knows it but me.

My abilities and limitations are a moving target and are an unknown quantity. I evaluate, mentally, what I can do, how long it will take, how I will feel at the end, and what else may I be able to do subsequently. My expectations always exceed my capabilities, especially, when it is later in the day. Even though I have learned to pace myself, and try to manage myself intelligently and realistically, not taking on more than I could ever possibly do, it is frustrating. I want to do more. I used to do more. I could do more were it not for the MS. I am compromised. I have to live with a disease that has reared up his ugly head like a dragon and has become a permanent unwelcome visitor in my body. I am a handicapped individual. I am eating right, I am on medication, I exercise, I function as a contributing member of my family, my employer, and my society. I try to enjoy life. I do what I can do, but not as much as I want, not as much as I used to be able to do.

And, no one knows it but me.

I shared this piece with several of fellow MS'ers, as I have endearingly learned to call them. They all said it described many familiar things they had felt, but didn't how to say it so eloquently or thoroughly. That was rewarding and reassuring that I had hit on key elements that many others out there were also experiencing.

"Steve," Janis said to me one night, "Why don't you try acupuncture. Maybe it will help you." I was willing to try anything if it had a possibility of helping me. I made an appointment the next day. That was the beginning of a new set of experiences with Dr. Stuart Zoll, Doctor of oriental medicine, and an acupuncture physician.

Our first meeting was just about explaining my needs, my limitations and what he thought he could do for me. I wanted to walk normally again. I didn't expect a cure for MS. I figured he might be able to work some kind of magic on my legs so that I could take the regular kinds of steps that I used to take. I wanted my stride back.

Dr. Zoll talked about chi, and energy and oriental philosophy. He said he had treated MS patients before. I was interested in his successes.

"When people with MS come in I tell them this – I can help, if your body is still strong and able enough to respond to the treatments. I have had success helping people with MS who walk in here. They still have feeling and some control over their muscles. These kinds of people I can help. The ones who are so far advanced that they can't move any limbs. Those people I don't have any luck with. I do think I can help you. Want to give it a try? All we can do is try. It might work, it might not. But, I would like to try. How about it?"

"OK. I'm game. Let's do it!"

For the next month, I took three treatments each week. Most of his pins went into my legs and feet, but two went into my stomach, two into each hand and one went into the very top of my head. He made a chart of their positions and did them the same way each time I came in. A session lasted about 45 minutes. After the pins were in, I lay quietly and rested until he came in to remove them which only took a few seconds.

In a week I noticed some improvement. In a month I saw quite a bit of improvement. I cut back to two sessions a week, and stayed on that schedule for six months. By then I was walking with a full stride. I was normal again in my walk. I still had MS. That fact did not change at all. But, I could walk again in my usual way. No baby steps.

Along with the pins, which I never felt, I took a variety of herbs and other natural items. Some I took were Bucco, Toxex, milk thistle, OPC, calcium with D. Over time he changed some of them to other things.

"Hey, Steve. Hold still." I was at work and my boss reached over my head into my hair. This looks like an acupuncture needle. Right?"

"Yep, thanks." He handed it to me.

I had one needle Dr. Zoll had inadvertently left in my head and didn't notice it. It had been there over two hours. Clear proof I couldn't feel any discomfort. I didn't notice it either.

I had a hair follicle test which showed I had a very high level of several heavy metals, Cadmium and Mercury being the two most out of range. Some of the agents I took were for detoxifying them, and they worked. By coincidence mercury was in the news papers and TV reports at that time. It seemed a lot of mercury was is found in salmon, not all salmon, but my eating salmon, which I did maybe once a week, may have contributed to my high mercury level, so I stopped eating salmon. Doing that and detoxifying my system brought my mercury level down.

I had several discussions about mercury with Janis. We cut out eating salmon for quite a while, but I had an interesting talk with my dentist, Dr. Garcia.

His mother has MS. She's had it for many years. Dr. Garcia and I had just met, but it was obvious I had a problem so we talked about it. I asked him his theory on mercury.

I looked around his open aired office. It was modern, warm, inviting. He was about my age. I had decided to change dentists to find someone closer to my work. I was losing a half day to go to my old one. My first impression was that he knew what he was doing and his staff was very friendly.

His mother and he had researched everything he could find about mercury. She wanted her mercury filling removed. He wasn't sure if it would help. She said do it so he did. He removed out all her old mercury fillings, taking painstaking care to capture the mercury safely as he took out each one and replaced them with amalgam fillings.

"What happened?" I was curious.

"She showed no improvement. None at all. Didn't matter one bit. Too bad, but she's just like she was before I did anything."

I decided I didn't think I would benefit either so my I told Janis I had decided to leave mine in just as they are. I was going to change my mind. Not until something was really conclusive.

I eventually backed off to just taking one acupuncture treatment a month, which was more for maintenance than a continuing of improving. I had definitely leveled off and was not seeing anything getting better than it already was. And then, after a year and a half, I stopped acupuncture altogether. It was a positive, painless, and interesting experience. It was worth trying and I am very happy with the results. It restored my full stride. It eliminated my taking the 8 to 10 inch steps that accompanied my getting tired and overheated. Although I walked with an impaired gait, at least I could stretch my legs to walk in the manner I was accustomed to before the MS started taking me over.

46

MY BOSS, A few MS folks I've met and my family knew I had MS. No one at work except my boss knew. Surely some had suspected I had something because it was getting harder to walk and pretend nothing was wrong. It became more and more obvious. I could sense the looks that others were giving me. I knew they knew something was wrong. I felt the stares and probably magnified them unrealistically. Since I knew what was going, I assumed they knew something, and just didn't want to mention it. It was so awkward. I didn't want to tell and they didn't want to ask. I was sure the people I worked with were uncomfortable not knowing how to approach me.

I decided to tell a few that I was close to and trusted, and let them tell the others. The grapevine travels fast. I didn't have to tell too many. The word would get out that I had MS. That wouldn't mean much to most of them, but it was time to open up to them.

When I finally gave into the idea that I would and could no longer hide my MS and that I would allow people to see me struggle with a little knowledge of why, something quite unexpected happened. Since that time I have been continually overwhelmed by the kindness of others who never cease in surprising me with their willingness to assist me. They open this door, they pick this box up, they carry that sack for me, it happens daily in a variety of situations. I did not know that the fabric of mankind could be so sincerely good in their unselfish efforts. I was afraid I would burden others with my difficulties. I found another side that I have never experienced before.

No matter how small the chore people I know and perfect strangers alike would rush and go to great lengths to offer a polite gesture in order to make my life a tiny bit easier. It happens so often now, I have come to accept it as if they felt it was their duty. I oblige them, however, because I think it makes them feel like they have done something admirable, and I wouldn't want to deny them the feeling. I graciously say "thank you," and smile as genuinely as I possibly can.

47

DON'T ASK ME HOW I FEEL – I HAVE MS

TO THE CASUAL, unknowing, well-wishing observer an MS person is just someone who is having a little difficulty. They think there is a problem like a sprained ankle, or an accident injury, or some other rational explanation as to why I am not walking with the same coordination as I used to, or as normal and customary as most other people who seem to manage walking with little effort. Or, maybe they see a part of my body which is stiff and not moving naturally. Or maybe they notice my head jerk or my eyes twitch. And they naively ask, "How are you feeling. Are you OK?" The full answer is nearly impossible to give, so I blurt out some expected, trite response. "I'm OK." Or "just a little tired today." They don't realize they only see the tip of the proverbial iceberg. If they could see the enormity of the invisible MS icebergs, they still wouldn't know what to say.

In the morning my gait is fairly normal, but my muscles are stiff and tense. My head is clear and, except for feeling a bit tired,

I really am OK, and as good as I will get all day long. By noon my gait and stride are shortened, my shoulders ache slightly, I might be experiencing a mild headache, and I need to sit down and rest for an hour. My legs feel tingly, my feet are throbbing, my hands tingle, also.

In the late afternoon I am feeling exhausted. It is hard to walk without falling. I grab for walls, doors, chairs and anything else handy to offer support. My headache is a little stronger, now. My legs are screaming with pain and weakness. The tingling in my hands has increased. I am feeling de-energized. I have lost speed of thought, reaction time, and perhaps some degree of rational judgment. I have to carefully read my notes, taken to buttress my waning short-term memory. I am feeling a bit out of control of the situation, however, I am helpless as to a solution, and therefore my overall sense of self-esteem and self-confidence is compromised. I am armed with the knowledge that my MS is incurable, and progressive, which is not very consoling. I am likely to be a bit curt, overly demanding, short-fused, loud and generally not very charming by this time of the day.

As I arrive home I stagger into the house. All I want to do is sit on the couch. All the details of the day are fuzzy, and I feel like I have forgotten something, but am not sure what it is. My feet and legs are now at a higher level of pain than at any time during the day. My shoulders are tight and in pain. My headache is in full throttle now. My vision may be a little blurry. My legs jump involuntarily as I lay on the couch. Each leg feels like low voltage electrical current is running through it. At other times it feels like little balls are wildly bouncing against the inside walls of my calves, similar to a game of Pong..

Throughout the day my body is in constant flux. It is acting like a sounding board by sending me signals about different locations in my body. It is reacting to my stress level, the activity of my MS, how much sleep I got the night before, how hot the temperature is, what I have eaten and many other conditions. My body is a laboratory experiment with external drugs and medications mixed with its own internal natural chemicals. It is subjected to related side effects and is constantly interplaying with normal biological systems.

My feelings are three-dimensional. They are based on location of the body, time of day, and degree of severity of a sensation. All three are independent variables. They all change throughout the day, every day without exception.

To offer an up-to-the-minute response of how I feel would take a while, and would require explanation, and answer the questioner. To the casual friendly observer it just isn't worth the effort. By the time I made a full and comprehensive response, some part of it would have changed, and it would then be inaccurate. Then, to be precise, I would have to offer revisions, and updates, and pretty soon I will have lost the inquirer altogether. They will now have wished they hadn't asked. And, I may not even be believed, as most of the physical sensations I feel cannot be witnessed externally. They are difficult to describe and even more difficult to be understood. Only an unfortunate few, who have personally experienced similar sensations, can truly empathize.

So, in the interest of time and good will, don't ask me how I feel, and I won't tell you. Instead, I'll just smile and say, "I'm OK. I'm just a little tired." But, I'll also be thinking to my unknowing inquirer, please realize that one should never judge a person based solely on outward appearances. MS masks itself and resides on the inside of the body, and a typical inclination to offer, "Oh, but you look so good, "will most often prove to be a very naïve and false generalized perspective.

48

PUBLIC ACCESS FOR THE HANDICAPPED

I HAVE, AT different times in my life, been on different sides of this issue. When one is healthy and normal, it is natural to only see life through the eyes of one who has no difficulties. It is too easy to underestimate, or be totally oblivious, to the enormous extra effort required of those who cannot move about as well as those who can.

I remember when ADA (Americans with Disabilities Act, Public Law 336 of the 101st Congress) was enacted July 26, 1990. I was working for Texaco, and I was in charge of operations and maintenance for 72 Texaco gas stations. All of them had to be converted to comply with the new law. Ramps to sidewalks had to constructed, restroom doors and front doors had to be widened, and many other similar changes. At the time, all I could see were the expenses. I thought rarely, if ever, were these changes ever going to be utilized by a handicapped person, so it was just a huge waste of money.

When I walked by a handicap parking space I wondered if it was really needed. I would see too many empty handicapped parking spots in front of many stores, and I thought to myself, "Why have so many when no one ever uses them?" And it really used to bother me when I would see someone get out of a car that was parked in a handicapped stall, and they appeared to walk quite normally. I would always look a second time to see if they actually had a permit to park there.

I was biased, and I admit it. Now that I am handicapped I have had my perspective turned 180 degrees, and I see through the eyes of the disabled person. Now I appreciate those ramps so my scooter or my wheelchair can climb from the pavement to the curb. I appreciate having the handicap parking close to the store, or the movies, so I don't have to go so far. And, I notice when they are all filled with other cars and I have to park farther away. Now I think sometimes they don't have enough spaces, not too few as I once thought.

I remember feeling guilty to park in the handicap space when I was still walking fairly well. There were times when I could walk a short distance with no pain, but when I had to walk further, it became very painful, and more so with each step. I'm sure people saw me walk a short way and thought, as I once did, that I did not deserve to park there. Those same people have no idea how much more pain I would have to endure if I parked further away, and the risk of falling would increase proportionately the farther I walked. Now that I walk with a cane and limp with my left leg, I guess I look like I need that handicapped parking. My awkward gait now seems to justify the privilege of parking closer to wherever I'm going. I no longer feel guilty, that is for sure.

The bottom line is that no one needs to look handicapped to qualify for a handicap permit. No one should presume to know the medical and physical limitations of another person. If a doctor says you are handicapped, you are handicapped. It's a shame how ignorant and short-sighted some people are. I readily confess I used to be one of them. It's just too bad I had to have MS to see the light. I hope others reading this will be as enlightened.

49

NUMBNESS VS TINGLY, TREMORS VS SPASMS

I WROTE THIS about 8 months after my diagnosis:

I came up with an idea to tell Janis how I was feeling at any given time in a way she might understand better what I was feeling. My legs are tingly, but about a #2 on a scale of 1 to 10. I am weaker than normal, but I have been up since 4:30 am, so I am probably tired from the lack of sleep. I just woke up then and could not go back to sleep, so I got up and did some organizing in my closet until it was time to get ready for work. At least the tingles aren't too bothersome right now.

My tingles are mostly in my legs, feet and arms and fingers. I used to get them more like #8's or higher, but I don't get them to that severe degree any more." I have learned a term for my sensations. It is called bilateral lower extremity paresthesias i.e. feels like electricity buzzing 24/7, sometimes better sometimes worse but always there.

Janis began asking me regularly how I was feeling. I replied with a number from 1 to 10. I think it helped us to convey my current condition better. When the number was high, there is less expectation that I could participate in whatever was happening right then.

If she'd ask how I was feeling, and I'd say 8, she got it. She kneow, without going into great detail that she might not understand, at that moment I was having a tough time.

Numbness vs tingly - it could be we are talking about the same thing. I can relate numbness to being really cold like when it is below zero outside. My hands are stiff and have no feeling. If you hit them with a hammer, it wouldn't hurt because I wouldn't feel any pain. In contrast, tingly is like electric needles lightly, mildly shocking, but no pain. More like when you sit on your hand for 10 minutes, and then you get up and your hand is asleep and it tingles until the circulation is restored. It also feels like that when you hit your funny bone (you elbow) just in the wrong place. I am using my own definitions, here. I don't know if MS – related terms differentiate them in the same way I do. The main thing about feeling tingly as opposed to being "asleep" is time. Feeling tingly can last for hours.

My rating system (scale 1 – 10) is arbitrary. It enables me to describe varying strengths of sensations. It helps to make comparisons. I can only tell when feeling A is stronger than feeling B. No one but me feels it, and you may feel something differently than I do, but my rating is a way to tell you that A, in my right foot for example, is relatively mild (say a #3) compared to B (say a #7), again in my right foot but much more intense.

When my ratings are low that is good. Low is closer to normal than high. Normal is not feeling any tingles at all. On my scale normal is zero. When ratings get up above 5 then I am getting uncomfortable, and the higher the number the more uncomfortable it becomes. I don't know what a 10 would feel like. I hope I never do.

I have both tremors and spasms, but not at the same time, fortunately. To me, spasms are when my leg, or arms, or shoulders jump involuntarily. Strangely, usually only one side jumps at a time. That is, I either have my left leg jumping or my right, but not at the same period of time. It can change an hour later to the other foot without warning, but only after some amount of calmness with no jumping.

My spasms occur late in the day, in the evening and at night when I am in bed. Since writing this I have more recently discovered tremors in the morning, especially when I get out of bed, when I get out of the shower, and when I put on my pants, and my shoes I have had spasms occur watching sports events or concerts, and I have wondered if seats without much padding set off my legs. But, I also get spasms sitting on my couch at home, so what I sit on may have nothing to do with it. When I get spasms I have found nothing that stops them, although stretching my calves, going up and down on my toes, does help. Changing positions doesn't help. I don't seem to notice them as much when I am walking, but that is not always an acceptable alternative.

At night is when spasms are the most bothersome. They are never painful. My leg just jerks as if I am trying to kick some invisible target in the air. Many are the times I have not been able to sleep because of leg spasms. Sometimes, I will wake up in the middle of the night and the spasms will start as soon as I am awake. I don't know if I have them while I am sleeping, however, I believe I do.

My tremors are quite different than spasms. With tremors my leg shakes as if I am toe-tapping the beat to a song. Again, the response is involuntary. The only way to stop the tremor in my leg is to change its position and weight distribution. When I was young, one of my early minor symptoms that now has become a regular, full-blown symptom, occurred when I stood on a ladder. My leg shakes terribly every time. However, now when I stand in certain positions, like when I stand one leg to put a shoe on the other one, I get tremors in my leg. Their occurrence is much more frequent and predictable. Tremors come to me always only one leg at a time, always the one that is holding the most weight.

I have learned to live with all these sensations – tingles, numbness, tremors and spasms. They are strange feelings that I have learned to accept as a part of my MS, and are a common part of the repertoire of symptoms of many who suffer from MS. I know now, having listened and read about all of them, that they are just mixed-up impulses, or signals, that are short circuited. My central nervous system (CSN) is behaving badly, but it is behaving. If I felt nothing at all, I would be worse, because that would mean that a nerve, or nerves, are severed, which is not repairable. The nerve(s) are dead. I prefer some feeling, even strange feelings, to no feelings whatsoever.

50

CONTINUING MY STORY things at my two jobs started piling up in ways I had no control over. My part-time job as a Manager for McDonalds became more demanding. My hours were increased due to keeping the store open longer. I had been working 5 PM to midnight on Friday, 3 PM to midnight on Saturday and the same on Sunday. Suddenly I was not getting out of there until 2 AM each night. I didn't get home and crawl into bed until about 3 AM.

The payroll and benefits manager at my day job was fired, and my boss gave me all of her responsibilities on top of the full time job I already had. I was the Facility Manager. I had oversight on all insurance programs. I was buying materials and supplies for the building. I was in charge of our safety program, worker's comp, compliance issues, negotiating new service contracts. I was also the security manager and Notary for the company. I also had to document and input daily rebate program details. With my new payroll and HR duties there wasn't enough time in a day. I was going in earlier, staying later, and going to the office on Saturdays to work extra six hours. I was working 100 hours a week.

It was hard to control my actions and reactions at both my jobs. I sought as many shortcuts as I could find. I lost my temper often, although I usually held it in check. When no one was around I slammed doors, cursed aloud, kicked waste baskets across the room and drove my car recklessly when bad drivers rudely passed me or drove too slowly.

I noticed the pain in my legs becoming unbearable which added to my anger. I didn't want to stand up, but I had to at McDonalds all during my shift. If I sat down and a customer or an employee needed me, I tensed up and met their beckoning with livid looks on my face. I wanted to be home resting. Why couldn't they leave me alone?

I began yelling at cars while driving. Fortunately, no one could hear me as the windows were raised, but I was not able to keep it inside. My road rage happened often.

"God, what a crazy driver you are!"

"How could you be so rude?"

"Why don't you let me in? I had my signal on! I flashed my lights. What's the matter with you, you turkey!"

"Don't cut me off!"

"Hey, can't you see I've got my turn signal light on?"

"Nice driving. What an idiot!"

"Unbelievable. Keep that up and you'll kill somebody. Just a matter of time, you clown."

If anybody had actually heard me, they would have wanted to run me off the road. Some of them seemed to be trying to do that anyway.

Although it was a software error from a new package not programmed properly, I paid about half of our 80 employees twice for one pay period, and most of it was electronically fed into their bank accounts. I discovered the error and, with the help of the payroll company we used, I got the errors reversed quickly, but my days on payroll were put to an end and I helped hire another person to take care the personnel duties.

I quit McDonalds. It was too much and I would have been fired myself if I'd been seen the way I was acting when I got so irate. I was pushing myself beyond my capabilities. I could do it, but not well enough to maintain my usual level of quality for all that I was doing. One of my best qualities was handling situations with a calm and clear thinking approach. I couldn't do that any longer. I needed to cut back and rest more. It was time. Past time no doubt.

It was at that point that my symptoms worsened. My body succumbed to the long hours of work, little sleep, and high demanding constant pressure. I don't know why I was reacting with so much anger. I just felt very tired, weak and in deep despair.

I think MS feeds on this kind of situation – pressured, stress, tired, and the rest. I was ripe for it to take me over.

51

MY DIET

MY DIET HAS evolved since my diagnosis and is now fairly set is its content, although it has gone through some fundamental changes since I began changing what I ate in response to my MS. I used to be guilty of the fast food temptations due mostly to the rapid pace of my life and having so little time. It was always much easier and faster to get something "to go" from a drive though window. It wasn't so much that I liked the food, but rather that it was quick and I needed the time. And eating all the free McDonalds meals came too easy. When I left my job there my diet began to improve.

Several years before the diagnosis I began to suspect diet was responsible for my headaches. Consuming foods and drinks that were sweet and loaded with sugar usually followed with a bad headache several hours later, or the next morning upon waking. Eating an assortment regularly of foods and drinks made it a challenge to determine which ones gave me the headaches and which ones my system easily accepted.

I began to develop a mental list which included chocolate, cakes and pies, fried foods, sodas, beer, candy, doughnuts, pastries, cookies, honey, maple syrup, chocolate, and many other fatty foods. I could no longer eat peanut butter, or jelly. Most salad dressings affected me. I reacted adversely to butter, and anything that was sautéed in it. I had to cut out the butter on my popcorn at the movies. Any food that had some kind of sauce on it or gravy gave me a headache.

The headache might kick in only after a few hours, or not until the next morning when I woke up. When it was the next morning I had to think about what I had eaten the day before. There was always something on my mental list that I could point to as being the culprit of my pain.

I had to stop eating processed foods. I used to love to eat potato chips and crackers. But, I always got a headache later, so I learned not to eat them. And, I trained myself to say "no" to them. Even natural fruits could be a problem for me. If I ate too many blueberries, or too much pineapple, I got a terrible headache. I can still sample a few, but I have to eat them sparingly.

What I just described was not easy and it did not happen all at one time. I had been collecting my list of "things not to eat" for many months. I also stopped eating red meat. No hamburgers, no cheeseburgers, no steaks. No meat in the lasagna or spaghetti, or tacos. But, then later I gave up pasta because of the sauces. I still ate grilled chicken breast and grilled fish as my protein, but still low on fat, and the rest of my diet became fresh fruits, fresh vegetables. I drank water and carrot juice. Lots of water!

When I found out that my mercury level was too high I adjusted my diet even more. I dropped the fish completely, presuming that the mercury in the fish passed on to me. My next test showed a drop in my mercury, so I have continued to avoid eating fish, except once in a great while. I have also given up eating cheese and dairy products.

I should mention I am not overweight. I have always maintained my weight at about 150 pounds and I am 5' 8" tall. I still wear the same size slacks and shirts I wore when I first was married. I exercise and I am healthy, except for the MS. I have become even healthier since all the diet changes. I never get sick. No flu bugs, no nausea, no colds, no sinus infections or cold sores.

An opinion I now have is that fresh foods do not need flavoring. They are delicious just as they come. It's laughable to me to say this, but when I go out to eat I notice that restaurants are all the same. They start with good food, but they add so much stuff to it to make it taste better they end up making it such that I can't eat it. For me a few quick delectable tastes are not worth hours of having a headache. So, I order my food plain. I have my salad with no dressing. I have my vegetables raw, with nothing on them. I have my entree served plain. And I drink water. It may not sound exciting, but it works for me.

I eat to replenish my body with nutrients that grow healthy cells. I no longer eat things because they taste good. I had to throw that concept out the window a long time ago. Now, I never get stuffed. I never feel like I need a nap after I have finished a meal. There are no highs or lows during the day.

A typical day goes like this for me:

Breakfast – 2 bananas, half a cantaloupe, water, and a few grapes.

Lunch – A heart of Romaine lettuce, carrots, raisins, 2 bananas, sunflower seeds, baby tomatoes, a sliced cucumber, and water.

Dinner – Romaine lettuce, broccoli, an orange or a slice of watermelon, an apple, carrot juice, spinach leaf, red cabbage, celery, cauliflower.

It is never exactly the same mix, but there are always several fruits, and several vegetables. I only drink carrot juice and water.

Recently, I have tried to stay with "organic." It is not always easy to find, and it is more expensive to buy, but I don't need any more pesticides in my system. I was exposed to all kinds of pesticides early in my life when I practically lived on the golf course. I was not aware of the potential risks of the chemicals that I came in contact with frequently. We used to buy fruit and vegetables from a fresh produce market. It was always fresh, but now I am not so sure how safe it was.

This diet has some variations as I eat different fruits and vegetables, and I am not on any regimented plan. I do stay far away from the foods that my body tends to reject. It just took a long time to listen and respond to what my body was telling me. I feel so much better, and I am convinced my MS is affecting me less because I am giving my system the right foods.

52

I MADE A trip to Chicago to see my sister, Sally, her husband, Dave, and their new baby. Sitting on the plane I was uncomfortable and began writing about my legs which were jumping with spasms and simmering in pain. It was a typical practice of mine to grab the barf bag in the seat compartment in front of me, pull down the table and write on it as my creative mind ran at its own pace, oblivious to the plane's noises.

SILENT LEGS

If my legs could sing, they'd be crying.
If my legs could yell, they'd be screaming.
The tone would be shrill,
The pitch would be high,
The sound would be cacophonous.
It would pierce the air like an arrow.
It would be vibrant with scattered discords.
It would be void of rhythm and cadence.
It would be pulsating with random strikes.

Resounding so loud it would be deafening.

It could wake you day or night without warning.

Echoing with its incessant, relentless noise.

If my legs were of color they'd be glowing,

Alive with ripples of burning red.

Controlled as if by an independent rheostat

Their hews vary in unpredictable brightness.

If my legs were capable of self-expression

They would tell you stories of pain and fatigue.

They could describe all sorts of sensations

Such as hot, cold, spasms and tingles.

They would mention electric-like pulses,

That can go on for hours and keep you up all night.

They would talk about poor balance and weakness.

They could explain about muscles swelling,

And tightness and constriction like chains.

They could show you the meaning of Drop Foot,

And of uncertainties ambulating on uneven surfaces -

Up hill, down hill, side hill, soft turf, high grass,

Mud, sand, slippery terrain, ice and snow - they all offer additional balance and fatigue challenges while walking or standing.

At this moment my right leg feels as if it has golf ball

Sized water balloons playing pong on the inner leg walls, bouncing at oblique angles, always in motion.

At other times they resemble the feeling of animated bubbles boiling in water, rising rapidly or simmering slowly as they cool off.

On the inside my legs speak volumes

With an extensive lexicon of sensations.

On the outside my legs are totally mute.

The day after returning from Chicago I fell twice. Once in the yard, and once in the house in the bathroom.

Once I got the mail in the mailbox by the street. I turned to speak to Janis with mail in my hand, and ….PLOP.

Janis saw me fall.

No problem. I got right back up.

I fell again in the house. I told Janis, "When I'm tired, I have to just think about walking and not talk at the same time. I'll have to stop, answer you, and then begin again." If I hadn't turned around to talk to her I wouldn't have fallen. I've learned that much the hard way. Remembering is different story.

After 4 or 5 falls I told Janis I had to look back and figure out if there was any one thing they all had in common. "You know when I fell I was doing other things while I was walking. I was carrying something, and talking to someone, and thinking about something else, etc., etc. I guess my brain can't physically multi-task like before."

"Well, you have to think about that. I don't need a damaged husband. You've got enough other problems already."

Now, when I walk, especially when I am on steps, or at a curb, slick footing, uneven surfaces or other potentially dangerous places, I just walk. Period. I push everything else away in my mind until I come to a stop. I focus on one step at a time, safely. I have not fallen once since, when I remember to do it, so I know it works.

I have also started making a record of my falls to help me analyze if there are things I can learn to be safer in the future. When, where, what was I doing, what was I carrying, what was I thinking, what else may have contributed to why I fell that time – I note as much as I can about the incident. It is part of coping with the disease, and adjusting to meet my limitations. I call it my KISS method. Keep It Simple and Safe.

I have 45 minutes to commute to work each day, and I gave myself the task of trying to come up with as many things relating to MS, using the initials M.S. as I could think of.

It became a daily challenge to add to the list I had started. In a week I had about 50 and this is how many I have now:

WHAT MS STANDS FOR

53

MS STANDS FOR:

Major Synapses

Making (no) Sense

Making Sacrifices

Malevolent Sickness

Managing Syringes

Many Shots

Many Spasms

Many Stresses

Marginal Steps

Marital Separation

Marital Strain

Massive Surges

Maximum Slowness

Missed Steps

Mistaken Situations

Misunderstood Signs

Mixed Signals

Moderate Sight

Moderate Symptoms

Moments of Sadness

Monetary Siphoning

MonSter

More Sensitivity

More Sensitivity

More Sitting

More Sleeping

Maximum Stress

Meaningful Seminars

Measurably Significant

Medical Studies

Medically Screwed

Medically Speaking

Medication Salvation

Medicine Selection

Melancholy Scenarios

Memory Sluggish

Mentally Slower

Mentally Stressed

Minimal Satisfaction

Minimal Sleep

Minimal Standing

Minimum Speed

Minimum Stride

Minuscule Sexuality

Minor Sensations

Minor Situations

Minuscule Strength

Misdiagnosed Sickness

Miserable Situation

Mishaps and Scratches

More Struggles

More Study

More Stumbling

More Support

Morning Sickness

Mostly Sensory

Mostly Serious

Motion Sickness

Motor Skills

Moving Sideways

Moving Slower

MRI Screening

Much Scariness

Much Shuffling

Multiple Scars

Mumbling Speech

Muscle Soreness

Muscle Spasms

Muscle Stiffness

Muscles Stinging

Muscular Sabotage

My Sadness

Myelin Sheath

Mysterious Sensations

54

THE ANSWER

ONCE THE DIAGNOSIS came I turned victim to my own unrelenting misery. Denial crossed over into bitterness and ran rampantly toward despair. Pain became a question, how much could I endure. No one was there to empathize, but, only there to criticize. Nothing helped to facilitate, or mitigate, but only there to tolerate. Answers came, unsettlingly. So much to doubt, so much to ask, so little news was comforting. So little offered hope, it sifted though my hands like holding sand. Could the unconquerable ever be conquered when all around me resounded clearly "no." Could I ever stand when all that I could ever understand was shaken beyond repair? Did anyone really care? And, there, right there, was where the answer lay. When I looked inside myself, I was only looking at myself, and was oblivious to the whole of me that makes my life complete. It is those around me who always surround me with lasting love divine. Their sacrifices over time belittle soundly the grievances of mine, and jolted me to come face to face with exactly who I am and what priorities have I defined. Bound in pure determination, tempered with anticipation, a certain level of acceptance has now been found. Knowing that I'm not alone has brought me light.

MY EVOLUTION

God works in mysterious ways. Although my life has changed dramatically, and my health has limited my ability to do physical activities as well as I once did, I see myself as evolving to a different level of understanding about myself and the world around me. There are approximately 400,000 people in the US who have MS. 100,000 males and 300,000 females, of all ages. Two and one half million people world wide. I have a certain bond with them now that wasn't there before my diagnosis.

I have begun to learn to experience how handicapped people survive. I actually always tried to ignore them because I did not know how to respond appropriately. Now, I see people doing that to me. The roles have reversed and have opened my eyes to a closer acceptance of my disability and those who are like me. I willingly exchange information about the disease with others.

There is inestimable value in knowing that one is not alone and there are many others out there who suffer as much or more than I do. All of us need help and hope. Being able to reach out and help others, or ask for help, brings an important exchange into the fray, which can be valuable to both the giver and the learner.

I don't view this disease as sad. I don't blame anyone. I don't make excuses. I do continue to fight my MS by proper eating, exercise, medication, prayer, education, and not trying to over exert myself. I do what I can do. If I think I can do it safely, I will try to do it. I am positive in my attitude. It makes no sense to me to be anything different. I have met many wonderful people that would never have crossed my path if I have not been ill. I have seen people unselfishly help me that I would otherwise have never known. I have been challenged to do things that I used to take for granted, like climbing stairs, or getting dressed, or walking around a large store. My limits and capabilities have been reduced, so I am constantly testing their boundaries. I have learned to cope with a myriad of physical sensations, many of them quite uncomfortable, which are so uncommon I still search for words to describe them. There is a certain growth and feeling of accomplishment in these things now. Many simple things have now become more important to me, and I have a greater sense of appreciation in these simple things. And, I am becoming more and more thankful that I have the support surrounding me that allows me to function and adapt to my new life.

I have the knowledge of having lived with MS most of my life, yet, regardless of how pervasive it may have been I have still been ambulatory and function reasonably normally. I am, indeed, fortunate that I have been able to enjoy life fully all my life, engaging in most activities that all healthy people do. I am thankful for that. My heart goes out to those who have seeming been robbed of the opportunities afforded to me over the years. MS attacks many young people, and they may never know some of the joys I have had the good fortune to experience. MS is too cruel, too capricious and indiscriminative in many respects.

So, perhaps, there is a trade-off for me. One perspective for another. One set of skills for another. One kind of humility for another. One sense of value for another. Yes, indeed , I am evolving. I do not know where the end lies, and perhaps there is no end. But,

I am certain that I am changing in many ways, and that is not altogether a bad thing.

55

DUELING WITH MS

I've always done my very best,
I've done a lot I must confess:
To stay awake without much rest,
I push myself beyond excess.
But, now I face with much disdain,
A matter I cannot explain.
Forgive me if I sound insane,
There is no longer much to gain.
For now I surely must regress,
To when it started to progress,
My doctor could not even guess,
That I was suffering from MS.
At first I tried to hide in vain
The fact that I was in much pain.
Dismissing all that I would feign
Which I now know was most inane.
It was too fearful to address,
And though I tried to make it less,

I was too weak. I was a mess.
My only hope was to redress.
And, so I came to face my pain,
Accept that I would need a cane.
I joined with others in the main,
And learned the facts I could attain.
Determination was my vest,
As I would fight this cruel guest.
Who's come inside to build its nest,
And threaten me to be depressed.
I look to no one else to blame.
Accepting this has been so plain.
My fears I cast into the rain.
No longer is my life arcane.
I face head-on this endless quest,
And use the knowledge I've possessed.
I will succeed, this life-long test,
And stay the course I will attest.
And, so my life has been regained.
I'm in control and will remain.
My courage stays so I sustain
The life I know I can maintain.
I cope with all that was repressed,
I know that I am very blessed.
And now that it has been expressed,
I pray a cure for all the rest.
For those anew can spare the pain,
And cross the road without restrain.
And live a life without a cane.
Be gone the reasons to complain.

56

THE UNPREDICTABILITY OF MS

WITHOUT QUESTION MS is frustrating because it is so unpredictable. There is doubt in every part of it. There is uncertainty in pre-diagnosis – when you first manifest symptoms. There is uncertainty in diagnosis. There is uncertainty in treatment. And there is uncertainty in predicting the path that MS will take with each individual. My MS has been unpredictable for most of my life.

What I call pre-diagnosis is the span of time, which may be a short period or many years in development during which MS popped up in uncomfortable feelings in my legs when I was very young. I am quite sure MS played a part in my youth, but in the 1950's it would have been impossible to have been accurately diagnosed and correctly treated. There just were not the tools available to determine what is was, and FDA approved remedies for MS had not been discovered. I can't blame the medical or research community for overlooking my problem. My MS was probably latent or slowly moving through my body with the force of a silent whisper. My body was telling me that things were not right, but I was ill-prepared to understand their significance.

I managed to somehow survive most of it's ramifications for over 50 years, living in this pre-diagnosis stage, while it stayed within a relevant range that kept it from being so severe that I had cause for concern. In that respect I feel very fortunate as there are many out there who have suffered far more than I, and have had their lives changed radically at a much younger age.

Again, I was more fortunate than many who have become plagued with MS when needing help became apparent. I went to my first neurologist, who did not help me in treating the disease, but at least his initial diagnosis was correct. I have heard about and read about numerous men and women who were misdiagnosed and had to suffer greatly from the bad call. I have since learned to appreciate how difficult it is, in many cases, to definitively diagnose MS. There are so many variables, taking in to account that each person is different, and their symptoms are different, and that many different diseases elicit similar symptoms, that it makes the doctor's job very difficult to be certain. Some doctors are more familiar with MS than others and can better recognize what they are seeing.

There is no one test which conclusively confirms an MS diagnosis at this point. I believe we are still in the infancy stages of the knowledge pool of MS. As a case in point, there are now six FDA approved medications for treating MS, Betaseron, Avonex, Copaxone, Rebif, Tysabri, and Novantrone. The first one, Betaseron, came out in 1993, and prior to then there were none. Prior to science being applied to MS, doctors, in some cases, would have a person suspected of MS take a very hot bath, and observe the results. If the patient was especially tingly then it was a good chance that MS was present in the patient and that is how a diagnosis was delivered. I have been told that there are over 100 research projects devoted to learning more about MS. Science is in our favor. And the amount of money directed toward these projects increases each year. I am very hopeful that some day MS will be prevented, and will be effectively treated when it is found.

That said, the frustration remains today for all those who have, or think they have, the disease. In what I have seen, it takes one or more attacks before you can establish a track record that begins a history of MS development for a person. You don't know you have it until you have had it for a while and it has affected you such that you have to be examined. It is not like the flu, or measles, or AIDS, or a thousand other illnesses that a doctor will know right away what you have. Unfortunately, there are many other diseases that mimic MS in one way or another which makes it much more difficult to make a diagnosis certain.

The FDA approved medications have been approved because in large clinical tests using large numbers of people, there were certain positive affects overall. There is no certainty that a medication will work for any one individual. Even in the tests only a percentage of the test group had positive effects, but there were enough of them to have the medication approved. I will only say a person should read all they can about them and be educated in choices, and realize there can be side effects, some of which will go away in time. For some, the side effects will not be tolerable and other choices may be explored. Even after you think you know you have MS, the uncertainty of what to take and how will effect you only adds another layer of doubt.

There are no easy answers. Only trial and error. One step at a time. One person at a time.

57

A REVERSED PERSPECTIVE

BEING DIAGNOSED WITH MS and looking forward provides a completely different set of circumstances than dealing with active MS for several years and looking backwards in time to when the diagnosis was first given. My original fears have long since passed and have proven to be totally unrealized worries. I did not die, although there was a moment when I considered taking my life. I did not lose my job, however I did quit my extra part time job. I can still drive a car. I did not lose my family, or my self-respect, although I came precariously close to doing just that. I can still see. I can still think. I still have my sense of humor.

I can (although I usually use a cane) walk. I do not know how far I can walk, but I have learned to stay within safe limits so I will never be too far from being able to reach a destination. I do know now the exercising and proper eating has helped me to walk further than I could at the worst of my symptoms.

I realize that not all who have had the misfortune of being diagnosed with MS have had the same degree of success that I have had. Some have had all sorts of serious shortcomings – job firing, loss of family, loss of mobility, loss of income, loss of friends, and on and on. Again, MS is cruel and affects people in many different ways. Thus far, I consider myself not a casualty case. I've just have to make some major adjustments.

In my own way of thinking I consider myself handicapped, but not a cripple. I may never run, or jump, or punt a football, or ski, or skate, or hit a golf ball 300 yards, or do many of the activities requiring physical strength and skill that I once took for granted. But, I still get around. I still function. I still can accept and perform responsibilities. I can still interact with my environment and enjoy life. MS does not preclude me from being happy.

If I suddenly got much worse and was bed-ridden for life I may take a different perspective, but not necessarily. It's all about attitude. It's what's between the ears, not how well the legs, or arms or eyes are working. I have learned to see the good in just about anything. I have learned to accept myself as I am. I like myself, both on the bad days and the good ones.

I have assiduously gathered self-protecting skills to lessen my chances of falling, incurring accidents, making mistakes from forgetfulness, simply losing my grip over my daily life, and a number of other things which can only be attained through having incurred the experiences I have had to face. These skills of self-protection have become my new set of armor. I rely on them often.

For example, I take copious notes about anything that might be important. I carry spare keys in my wallet so I can never get locked out because I mislaid my keys. I am very cautious walking on soft ground. I am careful stepping over curbs and wet surfaces. I make myself remember things constantly, keeping my mind active and testing my memory to recall names, numbers, dates, etc. I play the piano and type to keep the fingers dexterous and challenge my brain to do it with the fewest amount of errors. Knowing that everything I do is subject to mistakes, I look for them because they are usually there somewhere. If ever I think there is a risk of falling, I plan where and how I will fall safely. I have had to put my ego in my pocket and realize I am not perfect, but I can function pretty well within my abilities. And I err on the side of caution and take extra care when it seems prudent to do so, which has not been my nature in the past.

The last three years have been both a period of learning and a time for adjustments. It called for a change in attitude which was instrumental in making my learning and adjusting possible. As long as I dwelled on how badly I felt, as long as I only wished that this was a short term condition and would soon go away, as long as I held on to the belief that everything should stay the same and resisted change, guess what? Nothing changed. My misery perpetuated.

I was incapable of seeing into the future. I would not have imagined myself writing about my MS two years hence. I could not have visualized myself as having a five year reservoir of MS - related experiences incomparable to anything I have previously known.

It is possible, perhaps plausible, that my writing about my MS has been healthy and therapeutic. I tried to put into words the incredible, strange sensations I was feeling. Doing that helped me to recognize subtle starts, stops, and variations and intensities of the tingles and pains and spasms. I learned to discern the difference of a headache caused by heat and a headache caused by sugar or fat intake. Instead of being the patient, I became the observer, the scientist, the scribe. It became important to focus on the data, and I couldn't just sit around having a pity-party, because I was locked in to the finer details of my own body's reactions. This change in perspective, examining how and what and where I was feeling, launched me over time from recognition to forming cause and effect relationships to solution discoveries.

I realize only too well that I am riding an MS train that is out of control. It can climb uphill or struggle downhill. It can stop and stay put in its tracks for who knows how long. It has no itinerary and no final destination. It can make random stops and can change course without notice at any time. I don't know if I will feel differently tomorrow, or about the same as today. But, I do know I will get through today and tomorrow, which is something I was very insecure about for many months after my diagnosis.

There is life after diagnosis! I possess now an inner strength, a self-confidence, that I had to find. It was there before, but it was so vastly shaken that I completely lost it. For many reasons, I have regained it. My family, my doctors, my friends and relatives, research, books, medications, seminars, a change in diet, acupuncture, exercise, vitamins, herbs, carrot juice, prayers from many sources, trial and error, and more – they all are contributors to the renewal of my confidence. I would not have succeeded without them. I am stronger, wiser, and I know myself better.

The wheel chair that Janis bought for stands in the corner. I haven't used it in a long time. It's a solemn reminder that screams only at me. I walk well enough with a cane not to need the wheel chair.

However, it's entirely up to me. If I go back and start eating a poor diet. If I stop exercising and let myself get weak from inactivity, then I will need it again. And next time I may not be able to recover from having to rely on it. I don't plan to allow that to happen. Ever. That's my promise to myself. A wheel chair remaining in the corner not being needed is as great a motivator as I can think of.

My family has been unbelievably supportive in my struggles. I have not conquered MS, but I have learned how to cope with it and not let it ruin my life. My methodology is similar to the way I used to play golf. On the course in my preparation for a shot I would check the wind, the distance, the lie, where I wanted the ball to land, and the best trajectory of flight. I would take notice of whether I was standing uphill or downhill. I thought about how the shot would feel. Then I chose the right club and made a successful shot because I had practiced that same shot many times before.

My approach to MS is the same. I look at my present situation. I recognize how I am feeling. What I feel, how strong it is and where I feel it, and what caused it all feed into my mind as variables to be sorted out. Based on my experience I will then take appropriate action to reduce and/or cope with it in the best possible way that I know works for me. I have been successful in applying this process, and it gives me added confidence. I no longer panic, or worry. I have "a club in my bag" for whatever MS throws my way. Most things I have seen and dealt with before, and if new ones come along I know I have the tools to face them.

58

PLATEAU

I HAVE BEEN for the last several months in a period of slight improvement. So imperceptible to be sure, but I feel that I am getting better little by little. Anyone watching me walk could not possibly come to that conclusion, as it is all hidden. It is what I feel and how I am able to move throughout the day, maintaining rather than losing my stamina. I have more energy, and a better attitude. Here is a current assessment of my "State of the Body" report (4/1/04) from my unique perspective. My left leg is much weaker than my right leg. It is difficult to put on my slacks in the morning because I cannot raise my left foot more than a few inches off the ground. I am not in any pain in my legs or arms. The tingly feelings are so mild I don't even notice them. My fatigue varies, but it does not fall precipitously downward as the day progresses, as it once did a few months ago. Rather, I increase my stamina somewhat by sitting and I have about as much energy at 6 pm as I do at 10 am, unless I have had a particularly rigorous day. And even then,

I am not as wiped out as before. I always have some energy in the evenings.

My headaches occurred less often and were less severe in strength. The spasms that used to shoot down my legs toward my feet were not happening as often, or last as long when they did appear. I had noticed they started when I was sitting or lying down, and often there was some pressure, or partial blockage of my circulation in my legs (such as sitting on a bleacher seat).

But, the spasms did not last for more than a few minutes and were not as intense. When they did occur, they only affected one side or the other for the full duration. In other words, I either had my right leg jumping, or my left. Never both at once. Never did they change in the middle of the evening. Whichever one it starts with, it stays with for that evening. They did not keep me awake anymore. Many nights I did not have them at all. I was eating mostly fruit and vegetables, and no fats, sugars, meats. I exercised, and more. I think there must be a connection, because these were the kind of things I had changed. They certainly must have been some of the reasons why I had gotten better.

I believe my semi-recovery was attributed to my dedication to a number of changes in my daily routine. I was on an exercise program which included the following: 150 knee bends every other night, 30 times raising up on my toes in between each 50 of the knee bends. I lifted a 5-lb weight in my car 300 - 400 times with my right arm, and 150 with my left, every other day. I would do as many push-ups as I could do without stopping every other night. I was up to 26-30 push-ups. My left arm was much weaker than my right, just like my legs.

In late December, 2003, I played golf with my son at Hilton Head, SC., and noticed that I could not shift my weight onto my left foot. A movement I did naturally and unconsciously I can no longer do even when I try to do it. I would get close to the bottom of my swing and I fell back on my right foot. I have played golf for almost 50 years and developed a good swing at an early age. Only recently has my swing changed unconsciously due to the weakness in my legs.

That summed up where I was physically at that time. I believed that it was important that I keep exercising and increasing my strength, especially in my legs. I had a conviction that the stronger my legs are, the longer I would be able to walk. The stronger my legs, the better balance I would have, as well. As I got older my upper leg strength would play a key part in being able to sit and get up from a sitting position in a chair, or car or a bed, or sitting on the toilet.

I wrote on 8/13/04: In the past several weeks I have been intently watching my left foot. I am unable to move the toes, except just barely the big toe. I honestly can't say if this just happened or was so gradual I missed noticing it. I have had trouble twisting my left ankle for a number of months, which makes it difficult for me to put on my left shoe and sock. I have to spear the opening of the sock with my foot as it swings forward while holding the sock. I then tilt my foot bending my knee way to the right and try to catch the opening of the shoe with my toes. Then I lean forward and push down jamming my foot into the shoe. It is a daily struggle, and it probably looks hilarious to watch. Or maybe I just look pitifully uncoordinated. I am sure I had less trouble donning my shoes when I was four years old. But, I get the job done no matter how much effort it takes.

I wrote on 8/25/04: I went to my neurologist about my left leg. She asked if I had back pains, or had injured my back, which

I had not, in both cases. She asked me to get two MRI's, one for my spine and one for my neck. She also gave me a prescription for Prednisone, but only for six days. Today is day number six and I do not feel any different. Perhaps it is too early to see its affects. However, as time went by I believe it had no lasting affects of any kind.

One other note on this subject is that I now experience tremors in my left leg while putting on my shoe. Not all the time, but sometimes. This is a rather new addition, as until recently tremors only occurred while I was standing on a ladder. Now, sitting on a chair putting on my shoes can cause tremors in my left leg. Sitting on a couch, but leaning forward putting weight on my legs, will cause my legs to feel strained and fatigued. My legs feel better with no weight on them, or even better, raised and resting horizontally on the couch. As unbelievable as it might sound, I actually get tired while sitting.

I cannot raise or lower my foot, or swing it left or right. I do have complete feeling in all toes and the left foot itself. However, I seem to have lost all motor control over it. I cannot make it move like I can the right one. I can only make my left big toe move slightly. That is all. I try to move my feet inside my shoe, and can feel slight pressure against its inner lining, but it is disappointingly almost negligible.

I attribute my limping to the weakness in my left leg, left foot and left toes. I simply cannot put much weight on that leg. I also believe that the weakness that I have is a continuation, in a more advanced stage, of the same general problems with dragging my left foot while jogging years ago, and experiencing tremors climbing a ladder when I was young. My left leg has shown signs of MS all along, and it has recently become worse.

59

BEYOND THE END

I AM ENDING this book at this point in time, because there is sufficient information enclosed and there needs to be some point where I say enough is enough. This book has spanned over five years in its compilation and is comprised of all the major events and topics elated to my MS, plus a few personal stories interjected just for added value. However, since life and MS are both unpredictable I am now in the early stages of confronting some new problems.

My left foot, which is the same one that has allowed me to experience first hand about tremors going all the way back to my early life, has taken another step, no pun intended, toward getting worse. It is the same left foot that I dragged when jogging. It is the same left foot that catches on the floor and makes it easy for me to fall. It is the same left foot that has been difficult to put a sock or a shoe on. It is the same left foot that has had one or more black and blue toes for several years because I clumsily kicked hard immovable objects like chairs, and doors, and steps with it, regrettable and erroneously blaming my loving wife Janis. My left foot has been a problem to contend with for a long time.

Only about two months go, I noticed that I was not able to wiggle my toes on my left foot. I could not move my ankle left or right, or up or down. The circulation is normal. I have complete feeling in my foot and toes, but I have lost control and now have no ability to make them move. This is Drop Foot in an advanced stage, I believe.

I sought solutions for this, but thus far I have not found anything that worked completely. I didn't want to wait until I find a solution to end this book, so I will mention my foot problem and let it go at that. Continually trying to move it, pushing my toes upward against the inside roof of my shoe, has allowed me over time to regain slight movement of my toes.

I took 16 hours of physical therapy in small groups dedicated exclusively to qualified MS patients, and sponsored by the local South Florida National Multiple Sclerosis chapter. All exercises were designed to strengthen the muscles that my MS had weakened, but not destroyed. I made a list of the exercises that were helpful:

PHYSICAL THERAPY MS EXERCISES

Exercises while sitting:
20 with each – right, then left
Lift Heel
Lift Toe
Lift Knee
Leg straight out, point to up
Knees close and open wide
Turn and twist at waist

Lean forward, stretch far out and touch floor

Reach out like holding a ball

Place a ball between the knees and push knees against the ball.

Standing at rail:

Stand on heels

Shallow slow knee bends

Pull leg straight back behind you

Lift hip

Lift knee

Leg out to side

Lying on back:

Raise one leg, sliding foot toward body, knee pointing up, pause and slide back down

Keeping head still, turn legs and body to the side

Make a bridge, lifting stomach upward, touching surface only with feet and arms.

Sitting:

With back against wall, angle leg outward straight to stretch leg muscles

There are many more not listed, but these were the ones done most often.

The physical therapist was extremely helpful and corrected me on many of the exercises I had been doing. She also made me aware I should be doing more repetitions with my weaker (left) side. Rather than further strengthening my stronger (right) arm and leg, she recommended I build more strength into the left (weaker) limbs, and do fewer lifts with the side that was already further developed. That made sense. Try to make them more equal.

I have dedicated myself to do at least 100 knee bends,

twice a week at night, more when I am able. And I do 20 – 30 toe lifts nightly. As painful as these exercises were in the initial stages, they have proved worth the effort. I believe my gait, my ability to walk, my balance, and the longevity of being able to walk have been positively influenced by the commitment to these exercises. It is possible I may be back in a wheel chair had I not been doing them regularly.

Keep in mind I started doing about 2, because that was all I could do, but I have built up the numbers as I got stronger. Not only can I do more repetitions, I can stand in place longer. I can walk a further distance. And I incur less pain in the process.

Additionally, I have experienced reduced numbers of occasions where leg spasms have occurred. I am sleeping better, and am just less annoyed by the jumping legs that seem to come to me many evenings. My spasms appear to be happening less and less as I my legs get stronger.

To an extent, an autobiography of sorts is ongoing and has no end until my life is ended. I certainly do not wish to wait that long to end the book. In fact, I may compile enough data and new experiences to write a sequel to this one. For that reason, I close now and just offer that I expect many changes for the better as I face this disease, and apply my own learning curve to better cope with whatever it throws at me. Science, attitude, faith, prayer, my loving family, exercise and good heath habits are all on my side. Who could possibly ask for more?

I went through a period of time where I seemed to fall often, yet each circumstance was different. At meetings and seminars I heard several times the advice was given to keep a log and record events to gather information to share with your doctor. I began to log my falls. I wrote down when, where, how I fell, and what I was going for each incident. I kept this log going for seven months to determine, if any, common threads could be revealed. I was clueless as it seemed no falls had much in the way of similarity.

The results were enlightening. It had been a very useful activity. What I learned was obvious once I had gathered enough data to see the pattern. In a mater of sense, as the expression goes, I was incapable of walking and chewing gum at the same time. I never fell when I was just walking. But, in contrast, I often fell when I was doing too many "other" things while I was walking. When I was carrying something, talking to another person, looking left or right, thinking about something, listening to someone – or any combination of several activities at once while I was walking – my brain could not assess and process all that stimuli and walk safely forward simultaneously. I was overloading my Central Nervous System, and I was too spread out in my thoughts to move my legs and feet while all these other distractions were going on.

Having realized this I had to discipline myself to not be distracted while I was walking. When all I think about is putting one foot in front of the next I walk without falling. It is that simple for me. OK. I do one or two things carefully sometimes while I am walking, like carrying a package or watching cars go by, but I am aware that I am vulnerable and give my walking extra concentration so that falling is minimized.

60

MS AS A BLESSING?

I HAVE COME to understand my life in a different way, and MS has become a good thing because I only see the good in it, and do not dwell on the bad. I have met many people with MS, wonderful people, whom I would have never met otherwise. I have a new perspective on being handicapped, which I did not have until after my diagnosis. I have become more appreciative of my family and all that they do for me.

I am a stronger person, in character, because I have faced and dealt with physical adversity. I know a lot more about myself and about MS. Although I cannot do many things I once did, I relish those things and am grateful for what I have had the opportunity to do before I started getting worse. My life is still good, and I am surrounded by caring people who are willing to help me if I need them. If I complain, I am the fool. MS has changed my life, but it has not destroyed it. Every day offers new challenges which I must face, but

I will face them and, God willing, I will celebrate the next day, and the day after that, and the day after....

It is not what is in my body, or my central nervous system that makes a difference, it is about what is in my mind and how I perceive life. And how I deal with what comes into it.

MS is a blessing to me, for all the reasons above. It has brought me far more than I had before. Actually, these were all things I already had, but it took MS to help me really see them in a new way. The way I should have seen them all along.

61

ATTITUDE

FOR ME, ATTITUDE is something I choose, and it is a fundamental part of my everyday life. It makes me get up in the morning, and it makes me prepare for the day. It makes me smile to those with whom I come in contact. It guides the words I use to speak and write all day long. It helps me to survive whatever fate throws at me on a daily basis. It makes me ask for help when I need it. It makes me plan for tomorrow, so I will be ready for it. It makes me laugh, and see humor in things around me. It makes me see the good in all things, even when it may not be completely good. Attitude is reflected in how I approach every moment that I confront. It is because of the attitude I have adopted that I am alive and enjoy life to my fullest given my limits. My attitude is void of regret, sorrow, negativity, excuse, self-deprecation, hate, damaging sarcasm, and depression. My attitude is filled with love, respect, appreciation, hope, desire, sharing and understanding.

I don't see a water glass as half empty or half full. I see the potential of what the water can do to make life better.

My attitude is my pallet and my life is painted by the colors I choose to use to paint myself and world around me. I try and keep my colors as bright as possible.

The End

Printed in the United States
128935LV00005B/43-72/P